W9-DFN-822

WIDE OPEN

My Adventures in
Polyamory, Open Marriage
& Loving on My Own Terms

GRACIE X

New Harbinger Publications, Inc.

Publisher's Note

Wide Open is a memoir that describes the life experiences of the author, who writes under the pseudonym Gracie X (and is sometimes identified as Grace in the text).

Real names are used in the Acknowledgments except for the individuals called "Hank," "Valerie," and "Oz," which are fictitious names.

All personal names in the Dedication and the main text are fictitious with the exception of Judy Jones (who is identified by her real first name in the main text), and the individual identified as Deb, who is also called by the nicknames Gentle Bear and Bear. All business names associated with the individual called "Susan" are fictitious. Berkeley, the setting where much of the story takes place, is used fictitiously in place of the actual setting.

For these reasons, any similarities between the fictitious names used in this book, as described above, and any real people and places are strictly coincidental.

Distributed in Canada by Raincoast Books

Copyright © 2015 by Gracie X
New Harbinger Publications, Inc.
5674 Shattuck Avenue
Oakland, CA 94609
www.newharbinger.com

Cover design by Amy Shoup; Acquired by Catharine Meyers; Edited by Marisa Solís

All Rights Reserved

Library of Congress Cataloging-in-Publication Data

X, Gracie.
  Wide open : my adventures in polyamory, open marriage, and loving on my own terms/ Gracie X ; foreword by Carol Queen.
    pages cm
    ISBN 978-1-62625-058-1 (paperback) -- ISBN 978-1-62625-059-8 (pdf-ebook) -- ISBN 978-1-62625-060-4 (epub) 1. X, Gracie. 2. Open marriage--United States. 3. Sexual freedom--United States. 4. Families--United States. I. Title.
  HQ980.5.U5X22 2015
  306.84--dc23
                                    2015010145

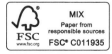

Printed in the United States of America

17   16   15

10   9   8   7   6   5   4   3   2   1   First printing

"Vulnerable and vivacious, *Wide Open* is a deeply personal, beautifully written tale of one woman's erotic journey to find herself and keep her family together. Gracie X bares her soul in this gripping memoir filled with pain and pleasure, growth, endings, and new beginnings. I couldn't put it down!"

—**Elisabeth Sheff**, author of *The Polyamorists Next Door: Inside Multiple-Partner Relationships and Families* (2014), and editor of *Stories from the Polycule: Real Life in Polyamorous Families* (2015)

"Gracie X has written an honest and engaging memoir about taking one of the biggest risks of her life—opening up her marriage despite warnings from friends and loved ones to not 'rock the boat' and her own fears. While honoring both her deep commitment to her husband and children and her reawakened sexuality, she shows us that, yes, we are capable of loving many people and receiving love back, as well as creating a marriage that is unique to our needs—a valuable lesson for all of us, whether polyamorous, monogamous, or monogamish."

—**Vicki Larson**, award-winning journalist and coauthor of *The New I Do: Reshaping Marriage for Skeptics, Realists and Rebels*

"For anyone who's curious about how to approach polyamory or open relationships with your partner, *Wide Open* is a must-read. Gracie X graciously lays out her complicated journey in a funny, honest, and relatable way that will inspire others to follow their heart. Redefining the family and relationship model is not an easy task; however, *Wide Open* gives you hope that through honest communication, emotional maturity, and patience, anything is possible."

—**Natalia Garcia**, director and creator of Showtime's *Polyamory: Married & Dating*

"I was moved by Gracie X as she shared a tender, passionate, and vulnerable memoir that inspires as it warns. This book is a must-read, authentic addition to the literature on open relationships and polyamory. As an intimacy counselor, I recommend her book for those who wish to experience the real-life joys, sorrows, challenges, and gifts of alternative relationship."

> —**Francesca Gentille**, contributing author of *The Marriage of Sex and Spirit*, radio host of "Sex: Tantra and Kama Sutra," and relationship and intimacy counselor

"This is a remarkable book. At a time when liberals and conservatives alike are embracing marriage and the nuclear family, Gracie X sends us a life raft—the bold chronicle of her quest to create a family configuration that works for her, her husband, new lover, and children. Gracie X is not only creative and brave—she is also a consummate storyteller. Be prepared for a riveting tale of her journey into intense new love while her marriage simultaneously evolves and realigns itself. For anyone weary from the dry, didactic tone of poly how-to books, this memoir provides a wealth of information about the triumphs and tribulations of exploring polyamory. And it is an indispensable resource for those seeking to forge a new way with their partners and families, expanding the bounds of even polyamory itself."

> —**Ann E. Tweedy**, poet and author of *Beleaguered Oases* (CreativePress 2010) and *White Out* (Green Fuse Poetic Arts 2013)

KITCHENER PUBLIC LIBRARY

3 9098 01533522 6

"To open her kimono and share how one woman and two families made sense of the paradox that is love, sex, family, intimacy, and honesty in our modern lives, is an act of tremendous courage and generosity. Her sassy, relatable, sexy truth-telling burns away the tarnish that convention can leave on our hearts. Even if our journeys look different than Gracie X's (as indeed they should), let us stand up and shout out: Viva the moxie of Gracie X to open her heart and her mouth. Say it, sister!"

—**LiYana Silver**, mentor for Women's Embodiment:
Bringing Your Feminine Genius to Life
(http://liyanasilver.com)

I wish to dedicate this book to
the warriors in service of love,
those who dare to love uniquely,
in their own way
with whomever they choose,
I toast you,
for the heart may be a lonely hunter
but she is also persistent and unrelenting
and there is no greater engine
than the calling song of the desirous heart.
To my children,
may you be warriors in the service of love,
seeking then finding all you need.
To Hank, for the perfect DNA and the great love.
To Valerie, for the willingness to go off road.
And forever to my beloved Oz,
you are my muse, my love, you are my muse…

Foreword

Carol Queen, PhD

Marriage is certainly in a state of flux nowadays. Some want in, some want out, and some want over the top, as though marriage was a wall you could scale to find a different garden on the other side. It speaks volumes, perhaps, that I—a conscientious marriage objector, listed on the Alternatives to Marriage website right there next to Beauvoir and Sartre, as well as an occasional officiant for marriage-minded couples who seek me out—should be tapped to write the introductory words for a book that is so much about marriage and its meaning. In the days of Old Marriage, I would not have been that guy.

But I work very close to the epicenter of what some call Modern Love. Yes, it was a terrific Bowie song, but now it's so much more: It's a movement of open-relationship believers, activists, and theorists, an army of lovers who refuse to believe that life's possibilities close off when they say "I do"—or who decide never to use those words at all, preferring, like Molly Bloom, to say. "Yes, yes, yes."

This movement goes by many names: polyamory or polyfidelity, open marriage or open relationship, Marriage 2.0. On one side of its vast net of life possibilities is a playful erotic culture; on another, a resurgent community (something like the communes and village life of yore) within which people raise their children in a nonnuclear fashion, thoroughly modern yet with roots that sink deeply into a way of life many of us postwar and new-century babies never knew till we re-created it. Some participants are creating family of choice because they can, and others because they must: LGBTQ partnerships are only at this very moment beginning to emerge from a world of alternative relationships, because "alternative" was the only possible flavor those relationships have been able to have.

Really, this movement consists of everyone but the players, the naysayers to love, and the married monogamists, for everyone in between those extremes of relationality has two things in common, however uncommonly they may express them: They are open to love and ongoing partnering of some sort, and they are open to having more than one such connection simultaneously.

Most of us (except maybe these peoples' kids) were raised in a zero-sum game as surely as the Cold War politics into which I fledged. You either were committed, or you weren't. You were true, or you were faithless. I was one of those people who wanted more than one person in my erotic and emotional world—maybe not both at once (though I've lived that way and valued it deeply), but at least potentially; I like triangles better than dyads, and always have. Maybe this is because I've acknowledged my own bisexuality since I was a teenager (though in a world of gender variation, that word seems more binary today than many of us find relevant, given our lived experience with more than just *men* and *women*); because I've always valued sexual curiosity and been certain I'd learn more from many than I did from one; or maybe it's because I watched my mother, trapped in a monogamous and gender-role-restrictive marriage, wither, starved of life's possibility. When I understood that this orientation on my part meant I'd be called a slut, I saw that word was meant to restrict me from experience I thought I had a right to explore—so it never really stung. If anything, it showed I'd already scaled the fence.

Being queer helped; it meant I was out of the box, maybe out of several boxes. Reading helped: I saw that historical moments that used to be called bohemian generally included a lot of relationship re-creation and experimentation, whether it centered around Frida and Diego or Natalie Barney and her many lovers, Bloomsbury or communes in the 1960s, the Beats or buffet flats, Paris before the war or the precious pre-AIDS renaissance of gay freedom. I learned that this way of loving had a history.

But that's my journey, and not the heart of the book you hold in your hands. When asked to represent, in just a few hundred words, Gracie X's journey—which is so thoroughly and individually *hers*, and so very illuminating of the cultural shifts that have roiled marriage over the past half century—I responded to several themes. Sex is part of the story; I was going to write sexual *freedom*, and that's true, but beneath that is simple desire for sex and erotic fulfillment, something too many people give up when they commit to one (sometimes not very compatible) lover. I am struck by Grace's insistence on loving commitment, growing together *and* apart, and the way she believes in working on her long-term marriage even as she looks for means to make that relationship morph into something new, a crucible in which new ingredients can be added. Mindfulness and communication are such powerful tools in a relationship that it's no wonder so many of us were never taught how to use them—see how much blessed havoc we can create when we do? And, of course, this singular story of Grace's is about parenting: making a safe and creative space for kids to have what they need to grow, a home in which all the members of the family have needs and must discover ways to align them—an amazing balancing act like a huge, poised Calder mobile.

This is a *woman's* story, though Grace chose to cocreate it with men—as lovers, partners, and coparents, her men have had to struggle, as she has, with bonds of expectation, especially the expectations of their community. We peek inside an alternative family whose engine for change is a woman, and whose perils weigh just as heavily on males as females. For there *are* perils in choosing to live your life outside the norm, though these are mostly enforced by those who stand inside the walls and peek unhappily over the edge.

—San Francisco, June 2014

Chapter 1

The idea actually wasn't my idea. My pal Sarah came up with it, and this was the nexus of my shock. Why the hell didn't I think of it? Was I losing my edge in suburban motherhood? Was I becoming a compliant, in-the-box thinker? When I heard the idea, I was suddenly struck that I had swallowed whole all the "rules" regarding marriage.

Several friends and I were attending a women's spirituality retreat in Mendocino, California, a couple of hours north of Berkeley. I took my ten-year-old daughter, Tallulah, with me as well; it was our yearly mother-daughter vacation of four days in the woods. Every year, we were so excited to go on our vacation that we packed a week early. I started coming to the camp when Tallulah was four years old. I was drawn there because the women were committed to themselves, to their evolution and unfolding, no matter what circumstance they found themselves in.

Attending that first retreat, I found myself in a circumstance fraught with the fear of losing my sense of self. After birthing Tallulah, I was stunned to discover myself in the desert of motherhood. I could see the ravaged bones of mothers all around me who hadn't made it. In the first few days of Tallulah's life, I was confused that something felt distinctly off. I loved my baby girl, and motherhood was filling me up in a way that nothing ever had. But it was as if an invisible noxious fume had floated into my home. I felt anxious and suddenly afraid of losing my essence and the unique heartbeat of who I was.

There were mirages everywhere. Smiling faces congratulated me on my new role as a mom, but when I spoke of my exhaustion they offered me poisoned water, subtle entreaties that it was now my *duty* to obliterate any need that might conflict with the overall well-being of my family. Although this was not the perspective of my husband, Hank, the attitude was so systemically pervasive that I felt like an outlier.

There were mothers who reflexively found refuge with each other. And mothers who had large supportive families and were genuinely revered. But in that first year, I saw other women sinking into the poisoned waters. The label *postpartum depression* took on new meaning, a clear misnomer—like the Romans diagnosing a Christian with anxiety disorder as he flailed wildly over the mouth of a hungry lion.

I knew instinctively that I would have to fight hard to continue to have a life that had me in the center of the frame. When I found the Mendocino retreat, it became my yearly salvation. The other women supported me in seeking methods of self-preservation. I now sought this not solely for myself; having birthed a daughter, it seemed imperative to role-model a path that kept me strong. At the weekend ritual, Tallulah would internalize a whole world where she was more than a workhorse or a Barbie doll; it was a place where she was revered for her strength and smarts.

At the retreat in Mendocino, we began to prepare for the Mother Crowning Ritual. Like every other year, it was sparsely attended. Apparently, mothering—even in the women's spiritual community—is a hard, sexless sell. As part of the ritual, women were divided into three stages of life: Maiden, Mother, and Crone. Crones were highly honored. You can cut in on any of the long food lines if you are over fifty-five and have been "Croned." Crones have exceptional clout in their longevity. And everyone loves a Maiden; they're so young and sporty—full of the eager questions and wildly arrogant assumptions about life that often mark youth. Tallulah was the youngest Maiden ever allowed at the retreat. She had about six "Aunties" teaching her meditation, archery, and goal mapping. I considered this long weekend part of her religious training.

At the ritual, Mothers were honored for their fertility and for their reigning place as the Queens of midlife (*yeah right*). There were three Mothers sitting around the circle making our Mother crowns for the upcoming ceremony. There wasn't anyone singing our song or tooting our horn—hell, we were *Mothers*. (There's plenty of lip service given to the great role of mother, but try pushing a baby carriage into a store your first month of motherhood, wielding it over the threshold as you struggle to keep open the door and watching as men glide right by you without a second glance. Who dives to help you? That's right, another frazzled, exhausted mother.)

We had tried to hard-sell the ritual to several women who didn't have kids and therefore technically were not mothers, yet were mothering large projects and businesses. But there were no takers. Just the word "mother" scared them off.

"But, ahh—I am not a mother," they would say.

Their looks seemed to harbor fear, as if by implying "mother" we were inferring "powerless, beaten-down hag." *Come on! Don't you want to create a ritual honoring the powerless, beaten-down hag in all of us? No?*

Three stalwart Mothers sat in a circle sewing little flowers and pinecones onto our wire crowns. Mimi, a fashionista who favors orange outfits, piped up and asked my friend Sarah about her "sexual pursuits." I was all ears because I knew that Sarah, like myself, had been married for more than twenty years and had two kids. Was her marriage as sexless as mine? Was she stepping out on her man? Hank and I felt mismatched sexually almost from the beginning, which frequently left me wanting more. We hadn't done the deed in a few months. I wasn't sure what Mimi was getting at, but there was way too much giddy excitement for her to be talking about Sarah's husband.

"Nothing has happened *yet*," Sarah giggled. Then she said that her husband, Matt, had agreed.

3

"What are you two talking about?" I asked, sewing a large hollow pod onto my crown.

Sarah went on to explain matter of factly that she had asked Matt to open up their marriage. She wanted to have sex with a woman, which she had never done but had always dreamed of. After a year of careful discussion and couple counseling he had agreed.

What? Say *what*?

At that moment the earth shifted and my world was altered. I literally sat speechless for many minutes, which was a highly rare state for me. Then my thoughts raced to the forbidden. I immediately started thinking, yet again, about my former Pilates client, Oz.

Oz, whose friendship I had ended at Hank's request. Both our spouses asked us not to have contact after they realized how close we had gotten. He lived a thirty-five-minute walk from my home, and our kids went to the same charter school near downtown Berkeley— still we attempted complete avoidance. But after three years of no contact punctuated by chance meetings, I was still thinking about him.

Our friendship changed my life. At first I couldn't imagine having much to say to him; Oz was so corporate and stiff. He was nine years my junior and seemed somewhat full of himself. But then I got to know him. I was usually the one asking the insightful questions. But he asked me questions too. His questions were from an engineering brain, pragmatic yet mystical—if that combination can be imagined. He had a facile, active mind, and his observations about me were unexpected and searing in their truth.

I felt so memorized, and by such a brilliant thinker. His conclusions were layered with kindness. He would shine a light on hidden parts of me that felt ugly, making them seem like gifts. Our conversations expanded my world—they felt like we were like taking a first-class voyage through the solar system, visiting planets, touching stars, taking breathtaking walks on the Moon. He adored me. To never see him again was equivalent to living in a tomb after meeting God on a mountaintop.

This love inspired me. Every time I sat down at my altar, I demanded (with a polite reverence) that the Universe bring me a miracle. I would not taint this great love with an affair, and I refused to hurt Hank or break up our family with a divorce. I would light my candles, write a little note, put it in my prayer box, and say, "I now turn this situation over to the Universe. I ask for a creative solution." I was asking a higher force smarter than me to send a new perspective. I would not act until I was presented with a better idea.

And here, right before me, channeled by my oh-so-ingenious friend, was my creative solution.

Later that day, while lying on my bed, I stared at the wood beams of my cabin roof. My heart was pounding wildly in my chest, my vulva starting to juice just thinking of Oz and the mere possibility that I might have sex with him. *What a brilliant idea! Why hadn't I thought of this myself?* I'd just ask my husband, Hank, very nicely, "Honey, would it be okay if I have sex with Oz?" And if he hesitated, I'd drop to my knees and whine, "Please, oh *please*. I'll do all the dishes for a month!"

The next morning we packed the car to leave. I made my last rounds of the tables covered with pagan crafts. Pagans have the best toys, the most opulent of ritual tools. Shopping at the witchy retreat was indeed a religious experience. I loved being surrounded by like-minded people in the craft whom I could casually question about a gemstone or oil they'd used in a ritual. Most people hear the word "witch" or "pagan" and assume I worship the devil or that I'll be abducting their family cat and frying her up for a sacrificial rite. This is so far from my experience of pagans, who create personal spells and rituals for the greater good.

No one at the retreat gave me the stink eye when I used the word "Goddess" to refer to the God force. I pray to Goddess as a reminder to myself that God has no gender. Why should the default position be male? However, I do appreciate the pluralism of paganism, which includes male deities. Splitting this massive higher intelligence into Gods and Goddesses makes it digestible to our little beings. I see my spiritual path as a constant integration of Goddess to achieve evolution and mastery in my life. This is why I love the word "witch," derived from the old English word "wit," meaning "to know." To know myself is my greatest path. All my magic—the ability to change my consciousness and life at will—derives from this place of knowing.

On the three-hour drive home I wondered if Goddess was working her magic with me, if there was a way to have Oz while keeping our families intact. Tallulah fell asleep in the backseat. I called Hank a couple of times to get a progress report on Merlin.

"I need fresh horses," Hank said.

They had made pancakes for breakfast and then played at the park, and now Merlin expected Mommy and Tula to be home. Hank handed Merlin the phone.

I heard his raspy voice say, "Mommy, I miss you."

I felt a tug on the invisible umbilical cord that never seems to entirely go away. I urgently wanted to be with him.

"Oh, sweetie, I miss you too. I have a present for you."

This lightened things up; Merlin became enlivened by the thought of future goods. I had some dinosaur stickers ready for this very moment; a Crone grandmother had put them on the treasure table available to take for free. Merlin was only five years old, and four days was an excruciatingly long time to be away from my Little Man.

When we pulled up in front of our house, Merlin was walking with Hank on the sidewalk. He ran to me and jumped into my arms. I held his wiry little body to my chest, breathing in his sweet smell.

We decided to walk a couple blocks to our favorite Mexican restaurant.

"How was your howling at the moon?" Hank asked as we walked.

"Fantastic," I replied, "I have so much to tell you."

At the restaurant, Tallulah pulled out all her loot to show Hank. At the retreat she was routinely showered with gifts. She proudly displayed the tigereye pendant around her neck and the gems from her pocket. I gave Merlin the dinosaur stickers—no dice. He wanted Tallulah's tigereye necklace. A brawl ensued. Merlin tipped over his apple juice. Hank and I tried to calm them. After five minutes of tears and shrieks, I took bold measures.

"Stop," I cried, "or no lollipops for dessert."

My kids sat at rapt attention. I never thought I'd bribe my kids with sugar. Before having kids, I considered that subpar parenting, but now that I had them I considered it a brilliant strategy.

"Can we please, Mom?"

They were quiet angels at the thought of no lollipops. I nodded consent. They ran off to get their lollipops from the waitress.

I met Hank's eyes across the table. We shook our heads and started to laugh.

"I really dislike children," Hank piped up in an English accent.

This was his stock line when things went south.

I gave my usual comeback also in a British lilt, "Is that so?"

Hank continued, "I find them quite tedious. Shall we send them away to boarding school?"

We both giggled.

Once, when I was pregnant with Tallulah, Hank went to get a bite to eat at a restaurant down the street from our house that catered to parents and children. He came home shaken. He described in detail a father who sliced his kid's hot dog. The kid went nuts screaming, "I can't eat it now!" Hank reported solemnly, "I think that little boy had some kind of brain damage." We were terrified that we'd also have a brain-damaged child. Then we had children and realized this was how normal kids behave.

We paid our bill and left the restaurant. We opened our front door. My suitcases from the trip were by the staircase. There was a pile of laundry by the washer that looked like a small mountain. I was increasingly overwhelmed as I walked through the house. After we got the kids settled in bed, Hank and I went downstairs. I told him some highlights of Tallulah being loved up by her Aunties. We had a bill or two we had to go over. We discussed our bloated mortgage, which I'd been trying to get modified. I suddenly felt exhausted and anxious, overwhelmed by the practical details of our life.

I told Hank I was having a bit of a tough reentry to my life. We hugged by the kitchen sink, then I went upstairs and crawled in bed with a glass of wine. My bed felt like a life raft—I wanted to float away on it. I flipped through the TV channels and found what I was looking for, a one-hour sensationalized news show. After a half hour I heard Hank coming up the stairs. He stood at the threshold of our bedroom.

"Watching some high-quality programming again, dear?"

Instantly shamed, I laughed. "I know, I know. It's embarrassing. You can feel superior that you watch mostly public television—when you aren't watching football."

Hank slightly smiled then nodded. He went downstairs, and I heard football on the living room TV. I knew I should be trying to connect with him, but I just wanted to zone out. The magic of being "between the worlds," connected to "infinite possibilities," had been smacked sideways by mundane life. Away from the inspiration of my tribe, the bright idea was starting to fade and a comfortable inertia was overcoming me.

The next morning we got the kids to school. I sat to check e-mails. I waded through the spam, repeatedly hitting delete. Then I noticed an e-mail from a friend in my business marketing group. She had sent me a link to another small-business owner's website. The subject column read, "You and Lily should meet and share resources." I opened the e-mail, clicked on the link, and gasped. The Universe was sending directions!

Redefining Monogamy was the name of the website. I perused every word. It described a process similar to what my friend Sarah was doing with her husband. It had quotes from couples who worked with Lily, who was not a certified therapist but a "counselor of innovative relationship styles." Couples were talking about doing "polyamory" and creating a new "vision for their relationship." With shaking hands I called Lily, and under the guise of networking I asked her to lunch the next day.

At noon, I was sitting at a café table on the sidewalk when Lily showed up. She was petite and strikingly lovely, with chocolaty doe eyes and dark wavy hair. She reminded me of the Lilith card in my tarot deck, which had a woman prowling like a tiger on a tree branch. But Lily had packaged herself for mainstream consumption: she wore stylish yet conservative clothes, not too much cleavage. I could read her thoughts: *You can't show up strutting how hot you are when selling open marriage. You'll be burned at the town square.*

We talked pleasantries for a while until I was ready to burst. After five minutes I told Lily that although I was interested in being referral partners for business, I was personally interested in what she was doing. I told her how much I loved my husband *and* how much I loved my children—*and how much I needed to get laid.* I explained to her that after twenty-five years, Hank was my best friend and my life mate. He held my hand during our home births. We created a life together that I had only dreamed of as a lonely child. If I could get his blessing, I wanted to open our marriage. I believed our love would remain constant even if we had sex with other people. My enthusiasm bordered on zealous optimism. I wasn't sipping the Kool-Aid—I was chugging it. This was exactly what I needed to create the massive transformation I dreamed of.

"I want to talk to Hank but I am not sure how to do it. I want him to understand how much I love him, but I want to have sex outside of our marriage. It isn't about anything being wrong with him—it's just so hard to imagine never having sex with another person."

"You are sort of a classic case in polyamory," Lily observed, "someone who is happily married but frustrated sexually. A person who values everything she has in her marriage but wants to have sex with other people." Lily gave me high marks. She said that the way I was thinking about how to talk to Hank was exactly the poly creed.

"Don't compare people," she advised, "express the devotion and love you have for your mate." And perhaps most important: "Go easy when explaining how you want to start dating again."

She said it sounded like I wanted "a primary/secondary situation." The primary partner would be Hank, who I was most strongly bonded with and legally married to. She explained that secondary partnerships are typically "relationships on the side" without the emotional, legal, or economic commitments of a primary relationship. I was excited—this would be great! Hank and I would get *secondary relationships*. It never once crossed my mind how complex this situation could be.

Lily went on to explain that there were as many ways to set up an open marriage as there were conventional marriages. Some people did "swinging," which was mainly focused on short-term, primarily sexual encounters. There was also "polyfidelity." This involved being faithfully exclusive to a triad or quad of lovers; for instance, you could be in love with your new lover and have him living upstairs while you and your husband lived downstairs. We also discussed one of the main poly principles: everyone must have full knowledge and be in agreement. Oz flashed into my mind—*What would his wife think if Oz asked to open their marriage?*

I told Lily I wanted to work with her. I needed to talk to Hank, but at this point I was a freight train of enthusiasm. Open marriage seemed like a great idea. Lily was excited to work with me. Then she told me she charged two hundred dollars an hour. This was a shocking setback. Apparently, opening your marriage was a pricy endeavor. But I was scrappy and determined. Immediately, I sold Lily on a Pilates trade for four sessions. Goddess was in the house—and magic was afoot.

Chapter 2

Our vows at the altar were about growing as artists and people. Our commitment to each other was to "evolve together" and to inspire each other to be our greatest selves. I was hoping that Hank would see open marriage as the next stage of evolution for us. Although, given our history, I wasn't entirely sure how he'd respond to the request.

When Hank and I first fell in love twenty-five years ago, we made an agreement. If one of us became attracted to another person, we would allow ourselves one sexual encounter. But after that we were to shut it down and bring our focus back to the relationship. Ours was not a well-thought-out plan. It was more a vague ideology with the underlying assumption that a one-nighter could be snuffed out easily without troubling the other person that it ever even happened. It was a barely scrutinized, "don't ask, don't tell" setup.

Five years into our relationship—enter Austin. I was getting ready to perform one of several plays I had written and toured the West Coast with. I had been writing plays and screenplays since moving to San Francisco. I was booked for a weekend run of a solo show made up of a series of surreal childhood flashbacks about my relationship with my mother. Austin was hired to do lights. I was standing center stage reciting my lines as we ran through the lighting check, and every time I needed a glass of ice water or to be guided back to my key light, Austin was there with his slim hips and wiry lean body. At five-foot-eight, he was four inches shorter than me. He gazed up at me with awestruck adoration, as if he were staring up at the Statue of Liberty for the first time—a really hot Statue of Liberty.

Instead of doing what a good married girl is supposed to do—say something like, "Why, Austin, my *husband* has a sweater just like yours"—I flirted outrageously, leaving him in the dark as to my relationship status. After the opening-night show over martinis at a nearby bar, I confessed that I was married. *But* I casually mentioned my agreement with my husband, our "one-time sex clause." Austin jumped at the offer.

Five weeks and a multitude of rolls in the hay later, I recognized that I could not fulfill my agreement with Hank. For the life of me, *I could not stop fucking Austin.* I decided I had to tell Hank what was going on. I hated myself for lying.

When I told Hank about Austin, he was very hurt. We "closed" our marriage and agreed to be sexually exclusive.

I contemplated this adventure during the next few weeks, and I came to a few conclusions. First, the loose "don't ask, don't tell" agreement Hank had proposed was a very pragmatic way of setting things up. Hank had instituted the occasional one-night stand. But I realized I didn't want *just* sex. I liked romance and a man who was interested in who I was. What I discovered with Austin was that if the sex, romance, and emotional connection were good, things were just getting started after one night. Stopping at that point would be like throwing a box of Godiva truffles in the trash. But when I brokered the deal with Hank as a twenty-three-year-old newlywed, I had little experience of myself in a relationship.

Apparently, Hank could not stop after one night either. After letting me swing in the wind for two months, hanging myself at my own self-created trial in front of all our friends, he confessed that he too had found it difficult to follow the rules.

I felt redeemed.

"So you had sex with someone and couldn't stop?" I blurted out.

But Hank refused to tell me any details when he spilled the beans during a weekend trip to wine country. All weekend long I interrogated him as we drove past majestic vineyards, soaked in hot tubs, ate a candlelit dinner. But I couldn't break him. The boy was smart. He knew I would have mind-fucked that information for years—*She was a size four? Are you saying you* like *petite women?* I was grateful he never told me any details.

After the Austin adventure our marriage remained closed for years, and that was good for me. I gave birth to both our children, and we hunkered down in our domestic nest. But as our kids came out of the baby stage, I longed for Hank and me to have more sex and romance together.

All around me I saw marriages at varying stages of passion. There were husbands who were highly sexual—but not with their wives. I had some female friends who were completely uninterested in sex— with husbands or anyone else. I saw marriages that were sexless but happy, couples who had moved into a place of being almost siblings or coparents. The questions that started to evolve for me were: *Can you be in a long-term relationship and have hot sex? How could Hank and I evolve our sex life so I could get more sex on a regular basis?*

The resounding thinking was that sex subsides in long-term relationships. But I was determined to have more. I wanted to make love as a way to play but also as an exploration of repressed, possibly taboo passions, the shadow aspects of our psyche that we could make safe together. I felt that there was more potential for us passion-wise.

I looked around my community. *Who had kids and a thriving sexy connection with their mate?* Some of my married friends candidly told me that they were *done* with the sexual and romantic part of their marriage. One friend with three kids told me that she loved her husband, he was a great provider, and she didn't care that they never had sex—she didn't care that "men no longer notice me." Her hormones had done their job and now she was focused elsewhere.

This attitude terrified me. It felt like falling into a pit of malaise and depression, like that bumper sticker "When all else fails, lower your standards." I actually read a self-help book around this time that tried to define sex as snuggling. Marriage "experts" were trying to tell me to get my snuggle on—*forget sex, lady!* If sex was having a long conversation about money and keeping our heads above water in this sinking economy that culminated in squeezing each other's hands, then I was getting laid regularly.

I refused to believe that more was not possible. *Who was still sexing it up in a long-term marriage or relationship?* I wanted to know what was working for them. I noticed among my friends with young kids that the people who fared best (by my standard of wanting family *and* sex) were those who had large, extended families helping to raise their children with them. Or the couples who had money to hire help that resembled a large, extended family. Although I didn't have that kind of budget, I made a plan to pay for a babysitter more often so we could have more date nights. I assumed we had scheduling problems. We just needed more time together.

Thus began the maddening, seemingly never-ending search for babysitters who were mature (enough to care for small children), affordable, and reliable—the winning triumvirate. There was a brief window when this crucible of attributes was met in a babysitter, because once they hit that first rite of passage—boyfriend or driver's license—I became like an old Hannah Montana CD: dispensable and boring. *Disrespect*—thine is a sixteen-year-old girl with a driver's permit and her first boy toy. Some nights I had to call more than ten babysitters. Half of them wouldn't even return my calls. I left pleading messages on their newly acquired cell phones.

"Can you just tell me if you are available…?"

When I did get them live, they'd inform me curtly, "Sorry, I can't. I am going to a Pink concert at the Warfield."

Teenage bitches. I had to hand out Starbucks gift cards and up the hourly pay to win a decent babysitter.

On one particular date night, the babysitter arrived and took our kids out on a walk and to dinner—more money. Unexpectedly, one of Hank's friends dropped by, and when I should have been getting pounded with my feet up in the air and my head thrown back while a stream of obscenities blissfully fell from my lips, I sat politely listening to the latest football stats on the 49ers. *I was in a domestic nightmare.* The moments ticked away, and then an hour later the kids returned to the house with the babysitter, her Starbucks gift card tucked into the front pocket of her svelte designer jeans.

I was beyond depressed. Having missed the sex window, Hank and I went out to dinner. What was striking was that Hank didn't seem all that bothered by the loss of potential nooky. He would have been howling had this been a loss of an hour to create art. At that moment I was too scared and depressed to contemplate why this was. When I opened the menu, a voice inside me said, *Order anything you want, old girl.* Indeed I felt old that night, like life was whizzing past me, spitting at me as it raced by in a glossy sports car.

A song from Tallulah's preschool rang in my ears: "The old gray mare she ain't what she used to be, ain't what she used to be, ain't what she used to be." Whoever wrote this song should be lynched by a posse of sex-starved wives. Was this the plight of the (*wince*) middle-aged? As I downed another glass of Shiraz and steadily overate my butter-laden mashed potatoes, the most disturbing fact was that Hank and I—although aligned in many ways—were not aligned in our intimacy needs. On that night what resurfaced from my subconscious was the daunting awareness of our sexual misattunement. For years I had stashed it in a drawer like an unpaid bill you don't have the money for and reckon you'll deal with later. On some level, my psyche had been wrestling with this matter until I could come up with a new plan. Things just kept puttering along in my life until one event or another would unfold and offer some insight into a better way.

One such event happened about a week before Christmas. Our marriage had been closed for more than ten years. Tallulah was seven and Merlin had just started preschool. I was cleaning up the living room and searching for stamps to mail some bills. I opened my desk drawer, but my stamp stash was gone. Damn. I looked around the room and saw Hank's aluminum box that passed as a briefcase. It was just the right size to carry all his pads and architectural notes; he had bought it at the local art store.

Good, I thought, *I know he'll have a stamp in it.*

I opened the box, not thinking twice about prying into what could be considered his personal space. I rifled through his papers and found a stamp.

But as I was putting the pile back into the box I spied what seemed to be a Christmas card. My eye zeroed in on the Polaroid glued to the front of the card. There was a voluptuous woman with bleached-blond hair; blue paint adorned her scantily dressed body, and she wore reindeer ears—the whole card had a performance-art feel to it. My hand reached for it like a magnet. I opened it and read, "Wonderful chatting with you last week. Love, Gabby."

I flipped back to the picture. Then I looked at the postage stamp; it was sent just a week ago from New York City. I knew who this woman was. I remembered her although I'd never met her or seen a picture of her. About ten years ago Hank's architecture firm won some awards. His was a pretty small operation, but an art student saw the press on his furniture and architectural designs and was wowed. She asked if he'd be interested in having her work as an intern for the summer. Hank interviewed her. Apparently, they had quite a bit of chemistry. The internship didn't work out because she had to go to Los Angeles for the summer, but they started writing e-mails to each other and got quite close until Hank ended it.

His last e-mail to her said something like, "I will happily dance at your wedding." A nice touch from a sultry Jewish boy. Hank told me about the e-mail late one night as we stood in the kitchen eating crackers and sipping cabernet. We'd hang out like this for hours, talking. At least once, I'd take a sip of wine, and then Hank would make me giggle so hard that I'd have to wave my hands for him to stop talking while I tried to control the muscles in my throat. Then when I finally swallowed I'd ride out the deep laugh.

I wasn't jealous. In fact I was kind of titillated. I was in the habit of thinking of Hank as Christ-like (another sexy Jewish guy). Hank was always so appropriate in his demeanor and response. He regulated his energy like he was pacing himself in a marathon. In this case the marathon was the longevity of marriage. His stride seemed to say, "I am not going to lose my balance over a small pebble in my path." A vision of Hank having a secret tryst, whispering sexily over the phone, popped into my head. My domestic messiah was being a bad frisky boy; it was exciting to see signs of his sexuality.

Hank had a great brand of sexy. He had a goatee and hair that spiked up in clumps randomly around his head. I'd seen women hit on him right in front of me. Once a barista asked, as she made him a latte, "Is that hair intentional? Or did you just roll out of bed after having fantastic sex?" Hank responded with a restrained but easy smile, his sexuality a slow, simmering flame. He was the stallion in the field quietly eating hay as the fillies in heat kicked up their hind legs in a flurry of zest around him. His response to the barista had a calm composure that fascinated me.

I looked at the Polaroid. There was only one way to find out what was actually going on. I pocketed the card. That night, I made one of Hank's favorite pasta dishes: primavera with mango sausage. We all sat down to eat. I poured the wine. Tallulah and Merlin talked about their day. At the end of the meal they asked to watch TV. I granted my consent. Hank and I sat at his Egg Table, an oval-shaped table made out of pine. It was a prototype that Hank had made ten years earlier, around the time of the e-mail affair with Gabby. It was one of many of his furniture prototypes in our home.

I asked Hank if he'd like more wine. He declined. I refilled my own glass. Hank leaned back in his chair. He was tired. It had been a long day. I sipped my wine. Then I put my hand in my pocket and felt the edge of Gabby's Christmas card. Hank was looking directly at me yet almost through me in weariness.

"Hey, I needed a stamp today." I started out the hungry cobra circling her prey. "I went into your briefcase box and found something interesting."

"Oh, yeah?" Hank stifled a small yawn.

I pulled the card out of my pocket like a sword out of my scabbard.

"What's this, babe?" I flashed it in front of his face; he focused on the card then flinched slightly. Now fully alert, he shifted in his chair then quickly took a breath, preparing for the duel at hand.

"Oh, yes. I was going to tell you about that." He laughed a small nervous exhale.

"So go ahead and tell me," I said pleasantly.

I was watching him closely. I could see by his body language that no great harm had been done. He had an attraction that he hadn't acted on. Christ scoped out Mary Magdalene's breasts. *He doesn't walk on water all the time.* He told me Gabby was coming to San Francisco to do a gallery show. He wanted to meet up with her when she was in town. I agreed to it. Oddly enough, it was giving me a vicarious contact high. I liked that the sex meters were rising, even if it was because of another woman.

Erotic energy is a precious elixir that risks evaporation in the onslaught of domestic life. *Nobody wants you to have sex.* Nobody supports your attempts at raucous, uninhibited passion. Your kids crawl into your bed every night like entitled land barons; they don't want you to have sex. Then there are all the bills and responsibilities; the PTA doesn't want you to have sex, and neither does PG&E or the IRS. Everyone wants you at work, pounding out a twelve- to fifteen-hour workday chock-full of responsibility and parenthood. It's one uphill slog until you may be lucky enough to have your life cut short by cancer or heart disease. After which you'll get a glowing eulogy about what a great sport you were.

But I still wanted to have sex. This was the first gasp of sexuality I'd seen on the home front in quite some time. I wanted more, even if the messenger was a body-painted bohemian in reindeer gear. My husband wanted to have a night out with a woman who made him feel sexy again. Good Goddess, don't walk—*run. Maybe this sex vibe will spread with contagious abandon.*

Two weeks later, Hank called me from his office. He just got an e-mail from Gabby. She was in the city.

"Can I meet her for a drink?"

"Sure," I said.

He headed for San Francisco at eight thirty, after we had plucked the kids from their bath and kissed them good night.

I grabbed the remote control and put on a grisly forensic show. I stretched out on our king-size bed glad to be free of the constant shaming from Hank and all my smug intellectual friends for watching these morbid shows. I was thrilled to be alone in my lowbrow habit. It wasn't the blood and violence I was after. *No,* I told myself defensively even though Hank wasn't around to judge me, *it was the intrigue, the strategy of the cops as they analyzed the crime and put the puzzle pieces together to nail the criminal.* After watching for a couple hours in pure hypnotic bliss, I turned out the lights. I tried to wait up for Hank but, surprisingly, at eleven thirty he wasn't home yet.

I dozed off. Later I rolled over, then looked at the clock. It was two a.m. and Hank still wasn't home. I was so surprised I grabbed my phone and dialed. No answer. I left a slightly sarcastic message.

"Hello? Perhaps you know me? We met at the altar several years ago for a small *marriage* ceremony?"

Hank had agreed to be home at midnight. It bothered me that he wasn't adhering to our agreement. It was one thing for him to get a little high; it was another if he started snorting it with no consideration to his promise. I dozed off again. I was awakened by the sound of the front door opening. I quickly sought the light of the digital clock: 3:00. *Oh, dude, you are so busted.* But I was too tired to initiate a confrontation. I rolled over feigning sleep, and soon I was slumbering again. In the morning it was all business as usual, nearly fifty mundane tasks to accomplish to get the kids off to school and prepare for the workday.

When Hank came back from dropping off the kids, he came into the dining room just as I was finishing my coffee.

"So?" I said.

"What?" he replied edgily.

"What happened last night?" I was curious more than angry.

"What are you talking about?" He delivered the line too quickly.

"Did you sleep with her?" I asked eagerly.

"Of course not."

He was starting to give off a Bill Clinton vibe, so I let it go.

It was an interesting turning point for me. I wasn't jealous and that surprised me. I was more interested in what was happening for Hank sexually. In so many ways we stimulated each other—as artists, as people, as parents—but our sexuality felt locked up. As happy as I was with our cozy domestic bliss, I was also increasingly uneasy. My head was jam-packed with illicit thoughts and fantasies that seemingly had no place in our carefully curated nest. I didn't know how to fix that. I wanted raw passion. I was fingering my honey pot daily—Technicolor sexcapades running nonstop through my brain like a preview to possible coming attractions. But these coming attractions didn't seem to have any place in our marriage. I wanted to unlock the cage and free the beast—but how?

Here was Hank's beast, and it was both a surprising and welcome relief—even though the beast had come out to play with someone else. I had been guiltily watching my beast run wild—if only in the domain of my mind—so it was a boon to me that Hank's beast had jumped the fence first. Yet now here he was struggling with the same sexual constraints. Was there a way this wildness could live in our domesticated world?

A few weeks later, when we were on a long walk in the hills, I decided to reopen the file. I wanted Hank to talk to me openly.

"Don't we have a great life?" I asked.

"Yes," he nodded.

I was feeling magnanimous. I felt genuinely blessed to have Hank and our kids, to be healthy on this beautiful day.

"Hey," I said as we ascended a particularly steep hill. "What happened that night with Gabby?" I peeked a glance at Hank and saw the internal quake.

"Nothing," he said sternly.

Right, I thought. I felt like one of those grizzled police detectives ready to interrogate the witness. We had another quarter mile up the steep incline, which somehow helped my interrogation.

"Babe," I said, smiling at him and slightly out of breath, "I know you made out with her. I am not going to get mad, just tell me, did you have sex or just make out?"

He looked bewildered, even alarmed. I could read his thoughts. Was I setting a huge mantrap for him? He was scared. I, by contrast, was calm. I wasn't setting a mantrap.

"Come on, just tell me. Did you have sex? I know you made out, just tell me."

I suddenly understood how those detectives broke down the criminal. They reassure them. They don't discuss jail time or any kind of punishment at all. They make the criminal feel completely understood, even justified. But in this case I was actually sincere.

Hank's eyes were shielded. He was really teetering. I knew he was thinking, *Shit, what's happening here? Am I going to be strung up by my balls in a matter of seconds?* He was scared.

"We just made out," he stated flatly.

We stopped at the crest of the hill, both breathing heavily, staring at each other, and then spontaneously we started giggling.

"Did you have fun?" I asked.

"What are you smoking?"

He was incredulous at my curious tone. I was surprised too. It was in this moment that we crept lightly into the forbidden land of acknowledging each other's separate erotic life. There were parts of Hank I had yet to know—and wanted to know. This could enliven our connection or kill it. I wanted to walk the edge of that border, in the hopes of creating more passion in our relationship.

It was in the same curious, hopeful spirit that I approached Hank about reopening our marriage on that fated night. I was skeptical about setting up another "don't ask, don't tell" agreement. Lily "the counselor of innovative relationship styles" had told me at our lunch meeting that some couples set things up that way. But I rejected the idea immediately. What excited me about polyamory was the honesty, the open acknowledgment that sexual attractions were normal, and the careful agreements made to preserve the primary relationship. For me, the "don't tell" policy housed some shame. I wanted to sit and talk with Hank openly. That was another fact I was sure of— lying to your man and best friend was a living hell I never wanted to experience again.

And now it seemed that the stars had aligned again. Since my epiphany at my witchy retreat, I had become jazzed again to recharge our marriage. After the Gabby episode, we had slid back into our normal relationship rhythm for two fairly uneventful years. But since coming back from Mendocino, a new pace of excitement was upon me.

It was ten thirty p.m. We had just watched the evening news. I had rehearsed Lily's pointers from our lunch just the day before. But instead of my planned speech, what came out was purely spontaneous. I leaned over to Hank's side of the bed where he had erected an insulating pillow barricade. Hank built it each night to protect him from the kick of any child who would invade our bed after midnight. I was barely able to contain my mounting elation.

"Babe," I said breathlessly, "tomorrow would you be into talking about opening up our marriage?"

He paused a moment, his eyebrows rose, and then "yes" was all he said.

The next morning, after the kids had been dropped at school, we sat down to talk. His first comment was, "Nice out-of-the-box thinking."

Then he asked, "Does this have to do with Oz?"

I was ready for this question, and I answered with edited honesty.

"Yes. Somewhat. But the truth is, I really would like to explore dating again and I am not focused on any one person." This was true. I was beginning to understand how badly I needed to be with someone who was excited to get me nude and whisper sweet nothings in my ear.

Hank agreed to my next step. He would do four sessions with Lily.

Chapter 3

It was the end of August. My marriage had been reopened for a few weeks—though describing it as "open" was perhaps a push. So far, Hank and I had had two sessions with Lily during which we started to explore what opening our marriage would look like. This did not change my internal state, which had become a fireball of excitement, gathering velocity by the second.

School was starting in two days. I had not seen Oz for months but he had texted me. In late July, he had sent a message asking if we could set up a "Same Time Next Year" arrangement. He said he "longed for a little grace—lowercase g concept" in his life and was hoping it could come by way of a "brief contact with Grace—uppercase G human concept." At the time, I had been puzzled as to how to proceed and what to answer.

In the movie *Same Time, Next Year*, two married people meet at a hotel once a year and carry on a secret affair that spans fifteen years. They never tell their spouses, and it does not disrupt their marriages. But I was unwilling to engage in anything that required subterfuge. I sat and prayed, asking for lowercase grace to step in and guide me. Two weeks after Oz's text, I got my answer at the spirituality retreat. I was waiting to talk to Oz after Hank and I had polished and refined our agreements. I finally responded to him in an e-mail that I had opened my marriage. It was the best I could do and, quite frankly, I thought it was a hell of a good response.

The next day, I stepped out my front door with Merlin. He was going to ride his tricycle around the neighborhood while I supplied moral support and cheerleading. We had traversed several blocks, and just as we were stepping off the curb to cross the street, Oz whizzed by in a baby-blue BMW roadster with his son in the front seat. My body accelerated to a warp speed of excitement. Oz gave a slight wave and then turned the car into the gas station. *Universe, thank you for your infinite blessings!* I was now forty feet away from Oz, who got out of the roadster to put air in the tires. Although it wasn't the place or the time to discuss my marriage, I couldn't deny the synchronicity of the moment—clearly the Universe was granting me an opportunity to talk to Oz.

Merlin and I steered his tricycle into the gas station. Oz's son, Liam, hollered for Merlin to get into the roadster, and they sat next to each other in the two bucket seats. Oz came up next to me, and I asked him about the sports car. His usual ride was a silver Fiat 500e, a pure electric plug-in car. Oz explained that he was test-driving it for the weekend. He was in line at work to get the roadster but said that he'd rather take cold cash for his retirement fund. I admired his lack of materialism. But he looked fine in the roadster. I commented on this. Electricity was in the air, but Oz seemed quite composed— considering what I'd e-mailed him yesterday. I mean, really? *How often does someone open their marriage in response to a request to have an affair?*

Finally I questioned, "Did you get my e-mail?"

He had not. Alright then, that explained his nonchalance.

I would tell him. But I needed grounding. I shifted my footing, taking a second to center myself. My body had been orbiting Earth at two hundred miles per hour, and I was gaining speed because I was also losing weight—I had barely eaten or slept in two weeks. I was a meteor catapulting through the atmosphere, confidently heading for my target.

I trembled as I opened my mouth, "Ever since I met you, or since we've become so close, I have been trying to find a way that I could have you and have my family too. I've been praying for a solution, and then I got this idea to open my marriage, and I asked Hank, and…"

Oz had on sleek sunglasses that echoed the roadster's sexy angles. I could sense him watching me closely, but I couldn't quite make out his eyes to gauge what he was feeling.

"… I opened my marriage so we could be together."

Dead silence.

I felt tingling at the back of my neck.

"Oh, Susan would never agree to that," Oz said quickly.

The meteorite hit Earth abruptly, then shattered into a million pieces. I felt light-headed. *I really haven't been eating enough.* I was running on fumes. Merlin started yelling—he and Liam were fighting over the stick shift. I leaned against the car. I suddenly felt ridiculous. Granted, nothing short of Oz throwing me in the BMW and revving off at top speed to the closest hotel would have sufficed, but this was an abysmal response. This was *no response.* I looked up at Oz. He was gorgeous, lean, and tall, and his movie-star sunglasses made him appear austere.

Describing my state of mind as "baffled" was putting it mildly. *Did he understand what I was offering?* I had found a way for us to be lovers without lying or potentially hurting our spouses! I was confused—I considered this a better solution than having an affair. Maybe he didn't understand how much I desired him. He had once told me that he was insecure about women finding him attractive, which was hard to believe given his Adonis good looks. Maybe he needed reassurance.

"I am going to have to grieve this," I said.

"Grieve what?" He was behaving very calmly.

"I've masturbated over you every day for two years. I'm going to have to let go of this dream of us being lovers."

If there's one thing I have learned about men over the years, it's that rare is the man who has a negative reaction to hearing that a woman masturbates over him. Not that I go around giving this information out like candy, but the few times I've told men that they were the star of my wet dreams—let's just say they weren't insulted.

But Oz remained still. Then I became mute. Perhaps that was why Oz started telling me about an e-mail he was crafting in which he had come to a similar place of not feeling ashamed for loving me. But I was feeling too dejected to listen. I was just thankful that the world had in it rich, fatty, deliciously dense foods, which I would be ingesting just as soon as I could grab my kid's tricycle and get away. I was profoundly confused. I grabbed Merlin and fled the scene.

An hour later, on a hike with my brother, I sat down exhausted on the trail. I told Munch (his nickname since childhood, Munchkin, because he's seven years my junior) that I didn't have enough fuel in my tank to keep going. I recounted what had just happened at the gas station. I felt almost humiliated that I had suggested my idea to Oz. It felt to me that Oz was rejecting me. Munch and I began to analyze the situation.

Oz and I had a complex history. For almost three years we'd longed for each other. A strictly professional relationship developed into an unexpected friendship, which became more intense as the months passed. Then one day, Oz called me from the wedding of one of his frat buddies. In a drunken reverie he confessed how much he longed for me. After his revelation I was filled with fear that we would do something rash and hurt our spouses—I slammed on the brakes. That conversation was followed by a two-year hiatus during which Oz and I worked on our marriages and generally avoided each other.

After his drunken reverie, Oz became almost puritanical around me. I could see this was his style—locking away, even denying, any conflicting feelings. Once, when I ran into him at school, I commented on how fit he looked (he had slimmed down—I had been his personal trainer, after all!). Afterward, he sent a bizarre, anonymous e-mail telling me that I had "broken the bylaws" by speaking to him and "not to comment on his body." My friends thought Oz was a bit of an oddball and socially awkward.

But his awkwardness inspired in me an even deeper sense of empathy for him. Although surrounded by a world of success, wealth, family, and other brilliant geek comrades, he seemed lonely. The recent "Same Time Next Year" text appeared to be a plaintive inquiry to have an affair. So it was jarring that he had responded so coolly at the gas station.

My brother and I broke into California therapy-speak. He suggested that perhaps I had been "triggered" by Oz's nonresponse. I agreed, saying I was "probably in a flashback," reliving past childhood wounds, particularly around my father. Munch suggested that maybe Oz "got scared and shut down." This helped a small bit. But I still felt supremely hurt and almost betrayed that Oz had barely considered my idea.

Munch drove me home as I mentally rehashed my conversation with Oz. When I got back, I ordered a large pepperoni pizza.

"How soon can you get it here?" I asked over the phone.

Forty-five minutes. What I really needed was a "Triage Pizzeria," where they rush the pizza to you by ambulance. In my haze of bitter embarrassment, I left a voice mail for Lily. I needed help badly.

Four hours later, I happened to check my e-mail and noticed two from Oz. I shivered with fear. I replied to him that I hadn't read his e-mails and to please "don't send any more," that I needed a "thirty-day time out." Then I received a third e-mail from Oz. This one I read.

> I know we're trying to detach, but first let me say you were so beautiful and vulnerable today. I am so honored that you think of me that way. And it was not my intention to make you feel rejected whatsoever. Right now, the concept of me and you allures and terrifies me, which is perhaps some of the energy you were picking up from me. I too need time to recombobulate, sit with my intellectual and emotional self, and try to figure out how to proceed.
>
> I will not contact you in any way until after Wed the 30th.

I love you so much,

Oz

So he had gotten afraid. This was reassuring, but his unpredictable nature still unnerved me. Another glass of Chardonnay and a large, gooey chocolate-chip cookie later, I was amazed at how I felt both jaunty and numb. I cavalierly decided to read Oz's e-mails, like a defeated boxer—beat up, bruised, but game.

His first e-mail opened with:

One thing I love about you is your amazing presence.

You've got to admit the boy was charming. I felt mollified. His second e-mail began with an acronym, something he would create as a memory aid to remember all the things he wanted to tell me—in the event of a possible chance meeting. CFSWALLOW listed all my amazing qualities in lengthy detail:

Courage (It's what you are, compared to timid old me.) Fun (You are so fun—but I'm scared of being extra-fun with you because of the fear that we'll end up stuck in thermal runaway. Wikipedia that, and tell me that engineering isn't cool.) Special (You make me feel special, which is something I don't have much experience with.) Worried (I've caught glimpses of you driving around in the Grace Mobile with a tense expression—I want to ease your worries.) Advice (Advice isn't quite the right word, but I need an A word so bear with me. I want to learn how to talk less about the moral failings of a person and do what you do—hold them in love and tell them how I think they can be a better person without it sounding like advice.) Loving (When we first met, you made me realize I was worthy of being loved. I didn't believe it before.) Learning (I learn so much from you. When we first stopped talking to each other, I was SO scared that you were the only one who could teach me spiritual and emotional things and that I had lost that forever.) O _____ (there's a void here. I don't have an O word for you...yet.) and Womanly (I've recently realized that, before I met you, I categorized the feminine with aesthetic beauty and the masculine with intellect, challenges, and excitement. But you, Grace, in addition to being beautiful, are also intellectual, challenging, and exciting in a very feminine way.)

I just love that in a person. Please! Do go on about my strengths. I felt now like the chocolate-chip goo in my cookie, until I was startled by this paragraph:

"Same Time Next Year." To me, the primary point of the movie was that they got to spend time together throughout their life...and then go back to their other life and people whom they also love. This is what I wish for us. The connection is so much more important than the affair, or lack thereof. I believe that the scriptwriters intended that. I mean the reason she was there originally was to go on a Christian religious retreat. He was there being an accountant for somebody's taxes. Accountants and nuns don't have affairs. They were there for another reason.

Was this guy for real? Accountants and nuns *invented* affairs.

Now I was mad. I had to respond. I could understand his being stunned by my proposal. But his words evoked some bad blood in our past history. The day after Oz had called me from the frat boy wedding, he wrote an e-mail saying he had to see me. He pleaded with me to just "break the rules" and "not tell our spouses." I could see how much he needed and missed me—but I also knew that if we were alone together, it would be impossible not to touch each other after our spoken revelations of attraction. So it was I that had maintained the boundaries, telling him I felt strongly that he needed to do therapy and work on his marriage. I even found him a therapist.

But later he confessed to me that he told his wife, Susan, that *I had wanted to have an affair with him and he had turned me down!*

What was even more interesting were the reactions of my friends and my brother. In an effort to process the episode, I told them what Oz had done. It split absolutely by gender as to how people saw this. All my female friends thought Oz was a schmuck and that the lie reflected on his character. But my brother and *even Hank* said, "Well, what could he do? *He was talking to his wife.* He had to blame it on you."

I had been forgiving in the past, understanding innately that Oz was not a bad soul and that he was clearly struggling with his feelings. But his current denial reminded me of the clergy in witch-burning times: in private declaring his lust and attempting seduction but sitting front row center at the public flaming.

Very well then, I decided as I finished reading Oz's latest e-mails. *The Bewitching Enchantress, the Evil Seductress will now emerge from the black lagoon of lasciviousness.*

I replied, referencing his librarian persona with the nickname that I had given to him after a few months of knowing him:

Oz, I've never understood the allure of the librarian. I was always baffled. "Are men turned on by how uptight the librarian is?" But the uptight quality is not the turn-on, although I find your introverted nature so sexy, it's this: You want to find whatever it is that will stop her from thinking about her Dewey decimal system. Oz, the idea, the challenge of making you moan inspires me. I want to find whatever it is that brings you to your knees, and gives you such ecstasy, that your top-knot blows right off your head. The idea of giving you pleasure turns me on.

I received this shivering response:

Grace,

There are seismic events and aftershocks running through my body right now, triggered by our conversation. I need to self-assess my feelings. Please wait until the 30th before communicating again with me.

How's that for a librarian response? :)

Oz

Nice. Mission accomplished. Seismic aftershocks—this meteorite had hit her target.

Chapter 4

At the mere age of twenty-three, I had the wizened heart of a forty-year-old—I was burned out on love. I had hung on for so many years, wanting to be loved. In college I was a bit of a promiscuous playgirl. But underneath my flirty exterior I was searching for love. As a child I tried to win the love of my psychologist father—who had divorced my mother when I was a baby.

When I was six years old, my mother started dating Ralph, a notorious criminal lawyer in Boston. I met Ralph one Sunday afternoon when he came to get my mother for a date. I set about to win his heart. The day of their June wedding, I was fully prepared to cash in my daddy chips and get the adoration of a male parent. After the wedding, my mother, sister, and I moved into the new house Ralph bought in a wealthy suburb of Boston a half hour away. My mother had our room wallpapered with a ballerina print and got us white twin princess beds from Jordan Marsh. Our first night in our new home, my sister and I were woken up by shouting, then slapping and more yelling; we sat shivering in our beds.

During the next several months this became our routine—we would be awakened in the night with the sounds of shouting and slapping. In the morning my mother would come and sit in our room. Pretty quickly my sister and I realized that Ralph was no prince. We repeatedly begged my mother to get a divorce. But my mother was snared, hooked on Ralph. She would stare off into space, her eyes blinking mechanically.

Ralph would describe his latest court cases at the dinner table: hit-and-run accidents, a little boy who lost his hand touching the top step of an escalator. He was always defending the store, or the person doing the hit-and-run. To my child's mind this struck me as odd. On the news there were reports of teenage-girl hitchhikers gone missing, then later found murdered. When a suspect was apprehended, he called Ralph for representation.

A year into their marriage my mother got pregnant. Ralph started picking boy names. When I asked him what he'd do if the baby was a girl, he smiled at me and said, "We simply won't love her." My sister and I got into a routine: as soon as Ralph returned from work, we would immediately go upstairs. We had become as notable as the muted striped wallpaper that lined the long hallway to our bedroom.

After the birth of my brother, Ralph started talking about how he was going to kill my sister and me. He would burst into our room in the middle of the night, drunk and yelling, insisting that he was throwing us out of "his house." My mother would be at his side, trying to pull him back into the hall. He would stand by our princess beds, his body rocking with rage, then describe our bloody bodies being found at the bottom of the stairs. Ralph yelled at us to get dressed so he could send us away to our grandmother's house. My sister would silently cry. But I would express my covert anger by becoming a little comedian, making jokes for my sister about selecting the perfect outfit for being thrown out of the house. My sister's spirit became more and more broken, and so perhaps it was my rebellious nature that caused Ralph to target me. One day Ralph showed up piss drunk at our summer day camp. I was walking up a dirt path when Ralph, who was hiding behind a tree, leaped out and tried to pummel me with a tire iron. Several counselors wrestled Ralph to the ground. The police were called, and I was delivered home to my mother, who divorced Ralph a month later. I have no memory of where I lived that month—it may have been with my grandmother.

Ralph and my mother were married for three years. It was her second and final marriage. Pictures of my mother before her two marriages show her baring movie-star teeth, her head tilted coquettishly to one side with a slightly nervous, glassy look in her eyes. She was a short-statured, curvaceous Venus with the frosty good looks of a Grace Kelly. After her last and final attempt at marriage, we lived permanently at my grandparents' eighteen-room old Colonial home, not far from where Paul Revere took his famous ride.

My mother's rage post-Ralph was almost indescribable. She had believed in the fairy tale wholeheartedly, but when her prince fractured her life, she woke up the disillusioned princess: fat, depressed, and really pissed off. She became a certified man-hater. During her graduate studies to become a social worker, she had idolized Freud. Post–failed marriages, she considered Freud a penis-obsessed cocaine freak. Her divorce was finalized in 1970, which was followed by a shrill decade in which she brandished her particular version of feminism. Men were banished from our world. They were mysterious, unavailable creatures in my childhood. I never visited my father, my mother did not date, my little brother was a child, and I stood back in fear of my friends' fathers.

At sixteen I sought out therapy because every time I liked a boy, if he liked me back, I had to fight the urge to run away from him. Upon hearing my history, my therapist suggested I find my father. I began to ponder his absence. *Who was my dad?* But my search for him ended in a disappointing visit in which he refused to help me with my college tuition. I was eighteen and my mother demanded that I ask him to pay for college at our first delicate meeting. He declined to help with tuition in a letter, in which he rationalized that I had refused to "accept his new family." I had told him that I wasn't ready to meet my stepsister (his daughter) right away.

At twenty-six, living independently from my mother, I sought him out again. I was determined to leave no stone unturned in my efforts to heal our rupture and finally have some semblance of a father-daughter relationship. During a weeklong Christmas visit I actually grew to like his Italian fatherly presence. Yet I needed to understand why he had not fought for me as a child. So I asked him to go to therapy. But much the same thing happened as did when I was sixteen. He withdrew in a veil of vague criticisms of my behavior and cut off all contact with me. Immediately afterward, I developed an unexplained throbbing pain in my first (root, a.k.a. buttocks) chakra. It lasted for months until a Chinese acupuncturist asked, as he was sticking me with needles, if anything having to do with my family had recently caused me grief—which started a three-day crying jag. When that ended, the pain in my tail finally subsided.

My experiences with my father and stepfather left me having little faith in men. In my mind, men either abandoned you or hurt you. I didn't think the words "nice" and "man" went together—until the night I met Hank.

After college, I moved to New York City and joined a lesbian theater troupe that performed regularly in the East Village. I had tried to be a lesbian. I was sometimes sexually attracted to women, and I felt fully aligned with lesbian culture, with one exception: I loved dick. However, I was highly ambivalent about the male person attached to the dick. I was resigned to make the best of my predicament. I decided I would get all my emotional sustenance from women and occasionally have sex with a man.

My friend Eve introduced me to Hank when he was visiting one weekend from Los Angeles. I arrived at the front door of her 1930s tenement apartment. Hank stood holding the door open. He had been sent downstairs by Eve to let me in—1930s tenements had no buzzers. Hank had wild hair and a nice-Jewish-boy quality crossed with a James Dean bad-boy angst. He was smoking a cigarette, and even though I vehemently disapproved of the habit, there was something alluring about the calm, sultry way he inhaled his last drag, then dropped the butt and rubbed out the last embers with the sole of his shoe.

As I walked through the door that he held open, he nodded and smiled at me. His hazel-green eyes were contained when he briefly met my gaze. Although I knew that all men were sexist brutes who would undermine and hurt you, a small voice whispered in me, *This is the man you've been searching for.*

I discounted the voice. We walked upstairs in silence. I wasn't going to get suckered into some romantic idiocy. We sat down and talked. Already I was fighting my attraction. Eve left to run an errand and I was alone with Hank for over an hour. At that time, I was around so many showboating actors working in the off-Broadway world that I expected Hank to launch into a self-promoting monologue of his feats. But instead he asked me about what kind of acting I did.

"Oh, I perform with a troupe in the Village. I haven't been able to get an agent yet."

"Is it hard to get an agent?"

"Well…"

Thoughts of my dismal, lonely life flooded me. Sometimes the only group I felt a part of was the crowd on the cross-town bus. Normally I would have put on an upbeat show focusing only on the positive. But instead I found myself saying slowly, "Everything is hard."

Hank laughed softly, "Everything is hard. I know about that."

His voice was smoothly sweet, like a thick patch of honey you'd find at the bottom of a warm cup of tea.

"So you're an architect in Los Angeles?"

"Yes. Have you ever been to LA?"

"I visited my cousin there when I was eighteen. I'm from Boston, and it was such a contrast. I never thought about how much history there is in Boston. I was kind of amazed how new everything felt there."

This was an understatement. I had been mortified by the amount of ugliness I saw in Los Angeles. There were poorly designed commercial strips that looked like they'd been put up less than a decade ago and would be torn down in the same amount of time. Hank seemed to sense everything I was thinking.

"I know. All the mini malls and apartments with the cottage cheese ceilings."

I laughed, "It was kind of ugly."

"There's no shortage of ugly in LA. Did your cousin take you to see any Frank Lloyd Wright houses? Los Angeles has some of the most beautiful buildings in the world."

Then he went on to describe several Frank Lloyd Wright houses in the Hollywood hills. The vividness of his words captured my attention. He had a sacred reverence as he described their beauty. He spoke of Frank Gehry's home in Santa Monica, how early on Gehry's neighbors complained that his iconoclastic designs were an eyesore in the neighborhood. "Eyesore?" Gehry had responded, then pointed at the boats latched to their banged-up pickup trucks in their driveways. Hank's description of architectural beauty started me imagining a completely different world that somehow I had missed on my visit.

"Do you have any siblings?"

I thought it was an odd question. I told him about my sister and brother.

"What about you?"

"My brother died five years ago," he said quietly.

"I am so sorry."

He nodded solemnly, his eyes moistened. It felt significant that he had steered the conversation and revealed this to me. Eve came home at that moment.

We started discussing the next morning's plans. Eve and I were going to an early-morning yoga class, and she was concerned because she had recently given up coffee. She explained that although she loved coffee, it was unhealthy. Eve and I vacillated between being avid purists, eating only macrobiotic foods, then succumbing to massive sugar binges.

Eve started a long monologue that sounded straight out of a Tennessee Williams play. In her lyrical New Orleans accent she discussed her latest passion: "the evils of coffee," the "pesticide-laden beans" that were likely to kill us all with their "toxic poisons." At the end of her impassioned rant, she lifted her palm, as if taking an oath to stop her own gush of words.

"Enough about how poisonous coffee is! Let's talk about something else. Hank, what are you doing tomorrow?"

Hank paused then said quietly, "Well, I thought I'd wake up early and get a bagel and a cup of poison."

I was unbearably smitten. He was funny but humble. Strong and masculine but gentle too. He epitomized what I am sure was meant when the word "gentleman" was coined. When Eve and I bid him good night and shut the door, I leaned against the wooden frame overcome with an attraction to Hank that felt so strong I was almost light-headed.

"I am in love," I declared to Eve, who looked up surprised.

"You should have told me! I would've asked him to sleep over," Eve exclaimed.

We tried to get Hank back for dinner the next night, but Eve couldn't find his phone number. He was returning to Los Angeles after the weekend. Dejected, I let it go, figuring a long-distance relationship wouldn't work out anyway. But a month later, Eve, depressed and fishing for attention, flipped through her little black book to make random calls. Hank was the only person she got live.

She asked him coyly, "Guess who is in love with you?"

A week later Hank wrote me a card. I responded, writing him nearly every day, starting a courtship that lasted six months and culminated with Hank moving to New York City. He arrived late at night to my apartment, declaring that he was finally here and would never go away. We have been together ever since.

After a few years of living in New York City, Hank wanted to return to California. I was glad to leave New York City's ball-busting, mean theater scene. Hank was a California boy. I had always imagined I would live in California. We decided to move to San Francisco. We had visited it for a weekend during our six-month courtship; I had fallen in love with the city's progressive history and offbeat personality.

Our first month in San Francisco we were driving downtown in Hank's ancient revamped Volkswagen bug when the clutch broke. I was immediately anxious, accustomed to my mother's high-pitched raging in the face of sudden mishap. In the world of my childhood, car troubles were a cause for major panic. Hank turned to me and caressed my knee as the car slowed to ten miles per hour and motorists whizzed by us, honking as they passed.

"It's okay, baby, this is not a crisis."

"Really?" I said, breathless.

"No, all this means is that we'll drive home in first gear and piss a lot of people off because we're not going fast. This isn't a big deal."

"What would qualify as a big deal?"

"When someone dies, that's a big deal."

Both of Hank's parents were Holocaust survivors. The rest of their entire families had been murdered in concentration camps, but somehow they had survived. Hank's brother was a successful businessman in Manhattan who had died of a drug overdose at the young age of twenty-six. Hank understood that darkness existed in the world. I could not have been with a man who did not understand the delicate balance of survival. We aided each other in the pursuit of wholeness. We told each other all our stories, no matter how hard they were to reveal. When Hank heard my stories he dubbed my childhood my own private Holocaust. I found Hank a support group modeled after the teachings in the book *Children of the Holocaust*. Hank learned about how the Holocaust and his parents' depression had affected him and his brother. Our love together was a powerful agent of healing.

When we were searching for apartments in San Francisco, Hank was interested in looking at a place on Fell Street adjacent to Golden Gate Park. When we got inside, we realized that it was overshadowed by trees, with northern light that left it feeling dark and gloomy to me.

"What do you think?" he asked.

"Well…" I hesitated.

We'd only been there a few minutes, but he really seemed to like it.

"I don't really like the lighting." I paused, "I think I'd feel depressed here."

At the time, depression was an unpredictable gray cloud that would waft into my life for weeks at a time.

"Oh, then let's get out of here."

His abruptness took me off guard.

"But, honey, if you like it, let's take it," I said.

We'd been searching for a few days and he really wanted to live by the park. He came over to me, took my hand, and looked into my face with a warm, amused twinkle in his eyes.

"Baby, why would I ever want to live in a place where you'd be depressed?"

In our first years together these moments stand out for me because they changed my paradigm for love. I spent my entire childhood living in a home where my despair and depression were huge, yet my parents did not seem to notice or care. Here was a man who didn't even want me to spend ten minutes in a place that would cause me pain.

Our chemistry together was inspiring. I started writing plays and acting at the local theaters. Hank got a job working with an architect, but after a year at this dead-end, "generic" firm, we decided Hank should quit his job. He would put all his energies into renovating the house we bought together, a dilapidated shack built around the time of the famous San Francisco earthquake. Hank speculated that it was built after the famous catastrophe as emergency housing; it was tiny, with a twenty-by-twenty footprint. We got it for ninety thousand dollars. When our friends helped us move in they joked that the place was so small we'd have to take turns being home.

We lived in the shack while renovating it. Two months into the demolition phase, with no toilet or shower, we started to fight like gerbils in a small cage. But a year and a half later, we felt victorious when we sold our renovated earthquake shack for $238,000. Our code and bond to support each other artistically had paid off too. When I attracted producers for my shows, Hank designed and built the sets.

Our friends, who at first thought we were nuts to buy the earthquake shack, now wanted to invest in Hank's future projects. Our close friend, Mike, unhappy working for the man as a corporate lawyer, asked if he could develop real estate ventures with Hank. They found a small plot of land across the bay in Berkeley, and Hank designed three houses on the lot. Mike and Hank hired a contractor to build the three spec houses.

At the last minute, Hank and I decided to buy and move into one of the houses. I had begun to supplement my meager art earnings with headhunting, a profession I had stumbled into. I was making an astonishingly high hourly wage that filled the wide financial gaps that were part of being an actor and playwright. This allowed us to buy our new home. We bought the house that Mike was worried would not sell quickly. The first two houses were in the typical craftsman style, but the third buffeted a busy street. Hank had designed it to respond to the four-lane avenue. It was reminiscent of a New York City loft with its industrial concrete floors, spacious twenty-foot ceilings, and windows in the loft-space living room. It stood in stark contrast to the quaint Berkeley neighborhood of California bungalows.

At first the neighbors treated us like interlopers. It was 1997, and there was a surplus of activity in the real estate market in California.

The small lot had been empty for ten years because of building code restrictions that put off the big developers. Neighbors had hoped for a dog park on the lot and were angered by the development. They saw us as wealthy investors, which couldn't have been further from the truth.

We were surprised that first Halloween when many trick-or-treaters and their parents politely asked to see inside, peering in from the front stoop, quietly exclaiming how beautiful our home was. Their kindness was gratifying, but we often felt mismatched to the affluent neighborhood. We had traded in our bohemian low-rent San Francisco neighborhood to be surrounded by couples pushing high-end strollers in their swanky fleece Patagonia on their way to vegan lunches. Hank missed our funky, arty neighbors in San Francisco. A few years after we'd moved in, two tax attorneys bought the house down the street; it had been renovated and sold for one million dollars, the first home on our block to cross the million-dollar mark. Hank and I met the couple and their new baby. When we got home we dubbed them "the adults." We still felt like irresponsible adolescents thrust into a grown-up world.

Ten years after moving into our modern, loftlike mansion, I was earning the bulk of our cash doing headhunting from home. After Tallulah was born, I stopped writing and took a hiatus from acting. When Merlin was born, I injured a muscle in my rotator cuff. I discovered Pilates and later set about getting certified. Hank and I transformed a room in our home for my gym, where I would build a clientele and business. With work that I loved and a family, I had achieved domestic bliss.

There are infamous moments that set a tone in any relationship. Mine came just a few weeks after Hank moved to New York City and we were living together. As a new lover often does, I could not keep my hands off him. When Hank entered the room I would move to him. I was mad about him. I'd watch him through my peripheral vision as we walked through the West Village, where we shared a tiny studio apartment. We'd hold hands and I'd take in his sultry air, calm demeanor, and languid walk. The boy turned me on.

One day, when we got home from breakfast at our favorite diner, he sat down. I kneeled in front of him and went to unzip his jeans when he said impatiently, "Every time I sit down you want to give me a blow job."

I had a split second in which I couldn't tell if he thought this was good or bad. But there was an overwhelmed annoyance in his tone. I was stung. Later, when I told my gay friend about it, he repeated Hank's words but with a completely different reading. "Girl! Every time he sits down you want to give him a blow job! You are a gay man trapped in a hot girl's body. That boy has won the straight-girl lottery. He should be thanking his lucky stars." But Hank was not thanking his lucky stars.

From the start we had mismatched sex drives. A tug-of-war began, which I am embarrassed to recount, I was not a good sport about. I would whine, complain, cajole, emotionally blackmail—all of which are very ineffective forms of foreplay. I wanted to feel irresistibly desired. I wanted Hank to rip my clothes off because he couldn't bear another moment without being inside me.

At the time, I felt deeply frustrated by our sexual mismatch. But I also thought of Hank as a superior male. He was not ruled by his sexuality. Hank was in direct contrast to my stepfather, who had strutted through our house, a male animal enraptured by my mother's beauty. Ralph and my mother's connection had a potent erotic charge. In my psyche, his violence and maleness, and strutting sexuality, were intertwined. I considered male sexuality to be dangerous.

Hank's response to his parents' trauma was to tamp down his passion and his needs. In my own style, I had a similar response to my trauma. Because of my history, I put my sexual escapades with highly libidinous men in a similar category to my stepfather, pigeon-holing them as dangerous in the long run. By my own design, these sexual men were relegated to peripheral flings and were separate from my life-building trajectory.

Part of my bonding with Hank was that we both shared the unconscious belief that unbridled sexuality was dangerous, thus we focused our relationship on emotional healing. My sexual tug-of-war with Hank reflected my own internal battle about passionate sex versus emotional safety. I now believe that *passionate sex can be healing and even create emotional safety*, but this was not my consciousness at the time.

Given that I felt I had only two opposing choices—sexuality or healing—I chose the latter. What I understand now is that I needed to do my own work in this area before I would be able to have both passion and healing—*at the same time, with any partner*. Hank provided a stable emotional foundation from which I built myself back, brick by brick. My mother was too mentally ill and my father was nonexistent. In many ways, Hank has been my first and most-lasting home base. When I was sad or overwhelmed with depression, which was a common occurrence in my twenties, Hank and I would snuggle, go to the movies, eat pasta, and nest. We made love, but it was not the glue that bound us together.

Tallulah's birth was the culmination of my healing in the area of family and safety. I moved from being the wounded child to being the source of a happy childhood. Oddly, motherhood, which has the power to desexualize many women (both hormonally and societally), became an instigator for me. Having achieved the ultimate in nesting, I felt both ready and urgent to grow with Hank sexually and create more eroticism together.

Again, I courted Hank sexually but from a more secure place this time. I brandished a seasoned, calm seduction—no longer would I play tug-of-war. I would not guilt-trip him into bed—which never worked anyway. I had discovered Tantra, which offered planned romantic interludes and solved our power struggle of my being the sole initiator. I signed us up for Tantra weekend workshops and classes. I wanted to wake us up better than we had ever been before. It felt urgent to resuscitate our sex life before the opportunity was lost forever in this new onslaught of parenting and domestic life.

But when I actively tried to woo Hank on a journey of sexual healing, what became apparent was that the more serious misalignment—beyond being out of sync in terms of sex drive—was in our investment and interest in growing together in the sexual and emotional arena. For me it became imperative, but for Hank it never reached that pitch of importance.

Chapter 5

My odyssey with Oz began with the act of advertising my Pilates business. Although I had not finished my advanced training, I decided to hang a sign on our front door and get some clients and experience. I was nervous about teaching Pilates without an advanced degree. Nonetheless, I plowed forward.

For several months I'd been practicing Pilates on my friends, my "Pilates guinea pigs," as Hank called them. I figured a small sign on my door was a passive yet clear signal to the Universe to send me a pig that would pay for my services. I decided to keep my rates low and be candid about my level of training.

I was *terrified*. In my mind, a mistake would be catastrophic. I approached becoming a Pilates instructor with the intensity one might expect of someone studying to be a brain surgeon. I was obsessively anxious that in my first experiences I'd nick a nerve or artery and my patient would be paralyzed for life.

A week after hanging up my shingle, I got an e-mail from a man. Osborn had just moved to my neighborhood from Monterey, where he had "a great personal trainer," he wrote. "I'd like to find another trainer to keep me honest."

I don't know what exactly it was about this e-mail that incapacitated me: the description of the unmatchable Monterey personal trainer or the plea for someone to "keep me honest." I didn't reply for days. Then I had a meeting with my manifestation coach, Deb, also known as Gentle Bear. When she heard I wasn't calling back a potential client, she folded her hands serenely over her round Buddha belly, leaned back in her rocking chair, smiled her Cheshire cat smile, and grilled, "You ask for clients, the Universe sends you a client, and you don't return his phone call? This is very interesting."

After a lengthy New Age interrogation about my contrary belief system causing me to impede success, I made a call to Osborn. With dread, I clutched the phone to my ear. I had in my mind a picture of who Osborn was. A man with a near-guru adoration to his last personal trainer, he would ply me with questions and then be disappointed by my inexperience. The whole imagined fantasy made me shudder.

I rallied my inner reserves as I heard the ringing of my phone. He picked up. I heard a deep, husky "hello." I introduced myself. The first thing I did was screw up his name. He corrected me quickly, unperturbed, enunciating it casually like a good corporate manager walking an underling through a new challenge.

"Oh, sorry," I mumbled, wondering how any parent could name their kid "Osborn," creating a sure destiny of ridicule and rigidity.

Osborn didn't engage in small talk. He almost immediately began asking very specific questions. He was particularly interested in my training style, which impressed me; he had clearly studied my website. He seemed very smart, very assured. We booked a session for the next day.

When the time drew near I was sick with fear. I had vacuumed, dusted, cleaned, and peeled a layer of my epidermis in preparation for his arrival. I was shaking like a leaf when the doorbell rang. Hank had just stepped out the front door to take the kids on a walk so that I'd be alone with my client. It was seven p.m. and my three-year-old, Merlin, had to be out of the house when I saw clients or he'd hang at my gym door crying for Mama.

My hands were shaking as I turned the doorknob, the internist preparing for her first brain surgery. *Oh, my Goddess, what if I nick an artery? What if I paralyze my patient?* Reeling with fear, I opened the front door. What I saw there confused me: Hank stood with Tallulah and Merlin next to a couple and their young red-haired son. Osborn turned to look at me; he was lackadaisical. It took me a second to realize that this was my new client. He had a tall quarterback build, vibrant green eyes, and tightly sheared blond hair, almost a crew cut. I would have noted how good looking he was but I was too worried that within the hour, due to my malpractice, he'd be carried out on a stretcher in a near comatose state.

Osborn explained that his wife wanted to see my gym. I nodded and said good-bye to Hank and the kids. I turned to lead them inside when their son darted past me and ran into my living room. He looked to be about five years old. Osborn followed his son, who was now playing with Merlin's toys in the far corner of our loft living room.

"Liam, we aren't going to play now," Osborn's voice was warm but firm.

His wife stepped inside beside me. She was attractively petite with long blond hair. She didn't smile or make small talk.

Who are these people? I thought, feeling mildly annoyed.

My nerves overtook me again as we walked upstairs to my gym. I led Osborn and his wife to the door of my gym. I stepped inside and Osborn followed, his hands on his hips as he surveyed the space. His wife stood at the doorway and peered inside. I couldn't read her expression, which was somewhat blank. She seemed to shrug; I imagined her thinking, "You call this a gym? It's a room with some yoga mats."

My Pilates equipment was on order and due the next week. I figured we'd do mat work that first session. My inner stage mother had shoved me forward to start my business—*now*—but standing there in the sparse room, I had another wave of nausea and anxiety. I was relieved when Osborn's wife left without reviling me for my lack of equipment. *Good Lilith, start the session!* an internal voice yelled at me. I looked at Osborn, who had an expectant look on his face.

I explained that the first Pilates session was somewhat tedious.

"Pilates asks you to learn a new way of moving," I said, "and it can feel confusing in the first few sessions."

Osborn nodded, very somber and receptive. He filled out a health form and I learned that he was an engineer. I asked him to lie on the yoga mat and showed him home position. His eyes were clear and focused. He made enough eye contact to show that he welcomed the challenge of learning a new system.

Two moments stand out about this first meeting. At one point I was lying next to Osborn on the yoga mat adjacent to his. I explained and then demonstrated a "functional exercise." A sudden feeling came over me, like we were lying next to each other in bed. *This is so intimate*, I thought. I noticed that Osborn averted his gaze when our eyes met. But the moment was fleeting, after which I continued with the session, teaching him a flexion exercise.

Then I launched into another of my rehearsed speeches.

"Weave your hands together, put them at the ridge of your skull at the occipital bone, float your head up, your elbows at a forty-five-degree angle, hold the position, then inhale and exhale three times."

Osborn watched me closely, paused, then said, "You explained that very well."

It startled me. I scanned his face. It was not so much a compliment as it was an observation. He nodded and smiled slightly, the executive approving of the subordinate's performance. My body shook as a new dose of cortisol cascaded into my bloodstream. Instantly, I knew he was wealthy, high on his company's totem pole; there was a confidence and prestige about him. I imagined him attending the most elite private schools and universities and graduating magna cum laude.

I felt like a small blemish on the chin of his world. I survived the rest of the session. Osborn told me he'd e-mail me. Two weeks later, hearing nothing, I knew he had compared me to Ms. Monterey and I had fallen short. But then three weeks later I got an e-mail asking for a permanent fixed schedule. I was surprised and excited to have my first steady, paying customer. Osborn requested Mondays at seven p.m. and Thursdays at five p.m., not the most convenient times for family life, but I e-mailed back affirmatively.

It took Osborn a while to align his work schedule to ours. He started coming regularly in July. Osborn arrived on time and worked hard. His shoulders were like concrete, his calves and hamstrings were also tight. Although he lacked flexibility, he had an inordinate amount of athletic prowess. He was only interested in exercises that challenged him. He needed big moves and a feeling he was being pushed to his limit.

That summer turned out to be extremely hot for the Bay Area. My gym faced south and the sun circled it all day. I'd start sweating as soon as Osborn entered the gym. It was both a nervous sweat and a natural response to the heat. I'd feel sticky in my armpits. Once or twice I had to straddle the Pilates barrel to demonstrate an exercise. As I carefully dismounted I'd check to see if there was a film of wetness from my crotch. Frequently there was a tiny lick of moisture, which I'd ignore, but I would quickly check Osborn's face to see if he registered it. Osborn wore a clement expression at these moments. If there was a film of perspiration on the equipment and we were about to share bodily fluids, no matter how miniscule, it didn't bother him. When I look back on this time I am struck by how completely absorbed I was in measuring up to my standards of the perfect health professional. I hardly registered Osborn as an attractive man—I was that focused on my hygiene and appropriate behavior.

I was grateful that Osborn didn't find fault in me as a trainer, or make note of my crotch sweat. I appreciated this in him. He himself was sweating quite a bit, but he had a robust air of acceptance. He'd grab a towel and mop his forehead, then proclaim loudly, "It's hot in here."

I admired his stoicism regarding my gym's climate.

However, his taciturn demeanor made me uneasy. I wasn't sure what to make of him. I usually developed an instant, easy rapport with people, but Osborn was so austere it made me feel standoffish.

His corporate job was clearly his priority and what consumed him. Oftentimes he'd e-mail that he'd gotten "pulled into work" and ask if we could meet later, pushing his five p.m. appointment to seven. I would grit my teeth and acquiesce. I hated working in the evenings and wanted to be done earlier than later so I could be with my kids. But I didn't want to lose his business.

It wasn't clear if he was working from home or commuting from Silicon Valley. Once, I had to call him to confirm when he was coming that evening. I dialed his number, getting a tight feeling in my stomach like Nixon's presidential aide must have felt as he approached him with an executive order to sign. *Would he snap at me? Would he be annoyed?* When Osborn picked up, I spoke quickly.

"Hi, it's Grace."

"Yes, what can I do for you?"

He wasn't cold, but it was obvious I was interrupting him and he wanted me to be fast. I had expected this. I inquired about the time we were meeting, he affirmed, and I got off the phone quickly. His remoteness made me even more curious as to what made him tick. So as I was setting up exercises I began asking casual questions. One sweltering evening, as I adjusted the bar for footwork, I asked if he'd had a fun weekend. The question seemed to make him uncomfortable.

"My wife and I went to Café West for dinner, is that what you mean?"

It was an interesting response, like he needed a categorical description of fun. I asked him if his wife was his best friend.

"I suppose so. Is that what you expected me to say?"

I was intrigued by his analyzing of what I might want him to say.

"I'm just curious," I answered. "I notice a lot of men say their wives are their best friend."

Osborn pondered my question while he adjusted his feet.

"I consider my wife to be my closest friend."

"That's great!" I said. There was something in his response that made me feel a pang of sadness for him.

At the end of the session it was check-writing time, a delicate moment. I'd nurture and bolster my client for a solid hour and now it was time for them to pay up. It felt both matter-of-fact and awkward. I needed to be paid, but under the circumstances one does not want to seem too rushed or eager. Osborn pulled out his checkbook.

Osborn asked, "How do you spell your last name again?"

I tossed out the name of the famous author who wrote children's fiction—with my same last name, save one consonant. I watched him as he wrote the check.

"I read all her books as a kid," I added.

Osborn paused from his check writing, "I did too."

"Oh, yeah?"

I was impressed. They were really girls' books.

Osborn continued, "The main character in the series was based on her. Isn't it funny, how if a character is based on the author she always seems to be so superior, so much smarter than all the other characters?"

I tittered—almost embarrassed. I'd written plays and screenplays wherein the main character (based on myself) had near-mythical powers and stunning beauty. Osborn tore the check from his register and handed it to me.

One night Osborn arrived very remote and quiet. Before I had time to ask him how he was doing, he said firmly, "Less talking." Then he proceeded to do the exercise I had just verbosely laid out. If he'd thrown a glass of cold water in my face, I couldn't have been more stunned. As every first-time Pilates instructor experiences, I had probably overexplained exercises using too much verbiage, and yet... *What an arrogant asshole*, I thought to myself.

I regained my composure quickly and vowed revenge. There are people you can piss off—your X-ray technician or your plumber—but don't piss off your personal trainer. For the next sixty minutes I put him through the toughest workout I could create that wouldn't tear a muscle or slip a disk. This was the night I dubbed him Oz, which I barked in a snide military tone (that I usually despised in other personal trainers) as he struggled to complete a massive set of pull-ups.

"Come on, Oz! Keep it up! Three more reps."

I was determined to knock him off his privileged Osborn ivory tower. But at the end of the session, mopping his brow with one of my pristine white towels, he said buoyantly, "Thank you. That was a great workout."

I felt wary of him from that point forward. I had learned from our brief conversations that he ran a large team of engineers. I felt sorry for the people who reported to him. But, in spite of myself, I respected the dedication he put into our workouts, even though he made me feel like a bombastic neophyte faking my way through my job.

After a few months of working with Oz, I considered him somewhat of a pill. He had the glossy good looks of a GQ model. There was a golden-boy quality about him—everything about him murmured of privilege. He lived about a dozen steep blocks away from my house, up in the Berkeley hills, where it seemed every vertical step increased one's income and house size. Oz wrote his checks from several different accounts: Vanguard, Ameritrade. I imagined pots of money that he leisurely pulled from to pay my meager fees.

One day he missed a session, a complete no-show. When I called him, he seemed bewildered as to who I was. I could hear his wife and little boy chattering happily in the background. I reminded him that he had a session at that very moment; he apologized quickly, said his wife just got home from a business trip, and that he had "completely forgotten" and wouldn't be coming.

Two days later, at the end of our session, when he pulled out his checkbook, I reminded him of my cancellation policy.

"You do know I have a twenty-four-hour cancellation policy?" I asked, surprised by my casual tone.

Oz was not particularly apologetic.

"So how much do I owe you?"

I flatly stated the number. I'd caved so many times with theater producers and production companies, working for little or no money. *I refuse to be a pushover*, I thought as Oz handed me his check.

In September, after five months of working with him, I stood gazing at myself in my bathroom mirror. I applied lipstick and blush, as I did for most occasions, and I studied my reflection. *I wonder what that guy Oz thinks of me?* I had steadily called him Oz after the affrontive night when he basically told me to "shut up and sing," secretly deriding him, since Osborn seemed the last person imaginable to make it over the rainbow. Still, I was curious. I had a vague feeling that he saw me as a specialized servant. But I wondered what he thought of me as a woman. I wasn't attracted to Oz, but I wanted to know if he found me attractive. He was nine years my junior, a young, sexy guy. *What did he think of me?* During our sessions I was so consumed with working to please his standards that I had not stepped back to consider what he might feel about me.

I imagined myself through Oz's eyes. During my poorest days I had cleaned houses for people to supplement my meager pay from acting gigs. Some people were really nice and personable, making me feel like just another human being who happened to be cleaning their home. There was one office in San Francisco that I cleaned in the evenings. Sometimes workers would be there late. They rarely looked at me. When I silently emptied their trash I felt like the lowest of the low. I understood how the eunuchs for royalty most have felt, the deep shame of losing the most primal ability to propagate, your purpose in life just to serve.

That was the feeling I got from Oz. I was his fitness eunuch—my purpose to serve his health, not speak too much, and certainly not to have any identity or sexuality. My sexuality was part of what I saw as my power in the world, so it was a bit humbling to have it completely negated. But it also felt like a relief not to be sexually objectified, as I had been when I worked as an actress. I was embarrassed having these musings about how Oz saw me as a woman. What did it matter?

One night, a few weeks after the "less talking" incident, followed by a series of quieter, more-intense training sessions, Oz arrived at my gym. Something felt off from the start of the session. His core wasn't firing when he tried to do leg pumps on the Pilates combination chair, an exercise that was usually quite achievable for him. I tried warming up his legs, but he was still off. His muscles were so tight that I suggested we release them. He was rolling out his iliotibial band on the myofascial log, proclaiming how much it hurt, when suddenly he stopped and slumped off the log.

"I should probably tell you what's going on."

"Okay," I said, off balance by his sudden openness.

I sat across from him on the yoga mat. Apparently his mother was going through a series of diagnostic tests for a serious digestive disorder. I'd had some clients who had the disorder. I asked a few questions and then told Oz what I knew about managing the disease, that it was livable and thankfully not fatal. I was struck by his deep concern; I guess everyone—even repressed engineers—have a soft spot for their mother.

He nodded somberly; he seemed relieved just to be talking. Then he stood up to do the leg pumps. His body was softer, less rigid. He did one perfect repetition, then another.

"Good work!" I exclaimed, looking up into his face.

I was about to say more but the words faded away. The intense vulnerability in his eyes took my breath away.

He's depressed—that's why he behaves like an arrogant asshole, I concluded to myself. I had an immediate sense that I could help him, that my particular gifts were exactly what he needed to learn. This would have been such a lovely Florence Nightingale vision filled with a pristine altruism—but in this lovely, guileless moment, my loins moistened and I developed a humongous crush. I was smitten.

This was not uncharted territory. I had been working for years to heal my "daddy crushes," as my friends and I deemed them. These crushes stemmed from a yearning for a father figure. When they first started in my twenties, I was looking for a platonic male mentor—a real daddy. But it never quite worked. The men who mentored me frequently wanted to cross the sexual line. I gave up on finding a real father figure. But what lingered was the longing for some elusive male validation. Ironically, my last few crushes were on younger men whom I had been mentoring. The paradox was that I refused to be sexual with these crushes and in fact wanted them to validate me— apart from the mutual attraction. This created a bizarre catch-22 for all parties. I was not surprised that with Oz's wealth and arrogance, he'd be the perfect next crush I'd attempt to win. I was prepared to ride the crush out for the next eight weeks, which was their typical duration.

I knew what was coming—eight weeks of the embarrassing predicament of being me. Observing myself made me cringe. I almost despised this needy part of me. She was about as dignified as those *Girls Gone Wild* videos, the ones that make you embarrassed to be female. When the ads came on TV I wanted to scream in feminist rage, *If you are going to flash your tits at least get some royalties!*

I was determined to get to the bottom of my neediness and finally resolve it. I did not take the situation very seriously. Oz seemed like a stable guy I could safely have a crush on without worries that he'd try to have sex with me. I needed time to untangle the conundrum of why I perpetually got these crushes.

But after eight weeks my crush was still thriving. All my methods, psychological and spiritual, were failing. I decided to decelerate my crush by integrating it into a potential friendship. My thinking was that if I got more male validation—keeping it platonic so as not to infringe on my marriage—the charge would fade. I pondered asking Oz to go on a walk. But I didn't quite trust myself. Was this just a rationalization to get into the cookie jar and stuff my face? I ran it by the small army of friends assigned to keep my mental health in order. I presented it something like this:

"You know the guy I have the crush on? After each session we chat, so I am not getting my cardio sessions because it bleeds into that time. What if I asked him to go on a walk? I'd get my cardio session and also…"

This is where things felt edgy.

"…He's like an appropriate librarian; we're both married, so the boundaries are clear. It could be an opportunity to have a platonic male friend, right?"

Miraculously they all signed off on it. Even Marc, my new therapist, said, "Let's see if you can get some of your emotional needs met through the friendship." I was stunned—like being handed the keys to the family Chevy after you'd crashed the Buick the week before. They all agreed that getting positive male attention might be just what the doctor ordered. I was excited but worried that they wouldn't have signed off if they'd truly seen the *real* me. Had I pulled a fast one: the Hunchback of Notre Dame dressed up in a pretty frock, a wisp of lip gloss barely masking her deeply deformed emotional hump?

Now mind you, I wasn't assured that Oz would even want to go on a walk with me. Oz seemed so busy and important. In contrast, I felt like Oliver Twist in the famous scene with his soup bowl extended: "Please sir, could I have some more?" But I was bold in the face of my vulnerability. I braced myself for Oz's gruff brush-off: "I couldn't possibly walk. I have a conference call from London in ten minutes!"

It was the end of the session. I watched Oz put on his shoes.

"I am going to take a walk in the hills—want to come?"

I flinched internally, my muscles tightening for the impending blow. I gave a final directive to myself—*appear casual!* Oz looked up. There was a one-second beat. Then, almost as if he were reaching out his hand from choppy waters as I extended mine from the lifeboat, he said simply, "Yes."

"Okay."

I was a bit off balance, so prepared for rejection I wasn't sure what to do next.

"Well," I giggled too loudly, "let me put on more clothes."

Did I really just say that? I galloped off to get a sweater, the ever-effusive teenage girl. A few minutes later we headed up the street, cars rushing by. We came to a fountain that served as a roundabout for six streets. I nodded toward the steepest hill, which I considered my personal StairMaster; on hot days it made me almost queasy to run up it. We traversed the incline, both starting to breathe heavily. Not a word was spoken. *We will survive this silence*, I thought.

After about fifteen minutes Oz pulled off his sweatshirt, exhaling heavily.

"This is vertical!"

I stopped too, hands on my hips, "What did you expect from a walk with your personal trainer?" We both giggled then continued the vertical ascent.

After a few miles we wound around the peak of the hill. I recognized the street name from Oz's checks. "Isn't this where you live?"

"That's my house there." He looked relieved to pause for a moment.

I looked to where he was pointing, at a large Tudor house sitting on the crest of the hill like a massive, regal dog surveying the bay.

"Nice house," I muttered, imaging the stunning 360-degree views from every window. Oz nodded, seeming to have missed the understatement.

We turned onto a hiking path leading into a redwood grove that thankfully began to wind downward.

There was another silence. Then organically we started finding topics. I told him about a dream I'd had recently.

Oz listened, then said pragmatically, "Dreams don't have enough reliable data. They're too random and frequently don't make sense."

"The night of my amniocentesis with Merlin, I was terrified he'd have some serious ailment—but a baby boy came to me in my dreams saying, 'Mama, I'll be just fine as soon as I get in your arms.'"

Oz was moved but still adamant. "Dreams still seem so random to me. Maybe your dreams are prophetic, but if I followed mine, I might become an ax murderer."

"It's the brain downloading the day's information that may have been lost in the mundane rush of life. You're still in control. I guess it comes down to, do you want more information or less information?"

Oz was silent for a long time. I guessed that he was seriously pondering my question. Or maybe he just thought I was a weird New Age hippy and wanted to drop the subject. I decided to let him be the one to break the silence, when he was ready.

Then, he said solemnly, "I like that—dreams hold information. As an engineer I will always choose more information."

It surprised me that I had said something that made him reassess his thinking. Oz was used to being around big brains. The last year that my mother was married to Ralph I became nearly mute in school and I was put in all the dummy math and reading groups. After moving back to my grandmother's house, the situation changed and I excelled at academics, but I wasn't back in terms of self-image. Oz's acknowledging my intelligence felt significant to me.

We started walking after every session. On one of our walks Oz confessed, "I am terrified to meditate." I suggested ways to take the "woo-woo" (incense and wind chimes) out of it.

"Just sit with yourself for five minutes and notice your heartbeat, your breathing."

A few days later he told me he'd done just that and wasn't frightened but bored.

"So you find yourself boring?"

This tickled him—he had to admit there was no one else there to be bored with.

"Aren't you curious to know yourself?" I inquired.

He chuckled, "Damn you! I accept the challenge. I will sit with my boring self."

On the next walk he confided that meditation had again become terrifying.

"No one in my life, including me, has ever been interested in how I feel."

This became one of our main sparring matches: an ongoing debate over the value of noticing emotions when it largely made Oz aware of his pain. Getting him to experience his pain was a hard sell, but during a particularly long walk—and debate—on mindfulness versus slogging in another hour of work, I asked:

"If your son Liam came to you and said he was in pain—would you just ignore him?"

He looked shaken by the question.

"No," he replied, "I'd do anything to help him."

"Don't you deserve the same?"

This was a conundrum for Oz, who was becoming increasingly aware that his primary measurement of his self-worth was his productivity. Although he would not concede to my value system—that he was so much more than what he produced—he was visibly moved by our conversations.

Oz quoted things I said, respectfully asking my opinion on a myriad of subjects: the body, spirituality, politics. I was getting some good stuff from a male pseudo-friend who was respectful and not trying to cross the line—it felt like real progress. My crush simmered down—yet still seemed like it could be on the verge of igniting at any moment—as I got respect and affection from him.

My sex drive had become an almost separate entity, outside of my marriage. I knew this was not good. My orientation to the problem was to fix myself. I had healed food issues, body issues, and many childhood wounds. I was confident I could heal *this*. My big problem was that I couldn't figure out what *this* was. *Why were all my usual methods to transform not working with these obsessive crushes?*

I was so wrapped up in managing my shame for wanting more— more passion, more sex, more affection—that I was taking total responsibility for my marriage dynamic. It never occurred to me that my wackiness might be a natural response to an imbalance of sexual needs and needs for attention. My thoughts around needing more were fossilized in a childhood perception of myself as flawed. I saw my crushes as evidence that I was still very wounded. What our culture glibly calls "low self-esteem" is simply the experience of doubting your truest self because you haven't experienced enough external validation and genuine love. Because I hadn't received many pats on the head from my parents, I was looking inward for my flaws when I should have been looking outward for what was not working in the societal box in which I'd stuffed marriage and family. I had been too inhibited to see the bigger picture.

Ending the crushes seemed dependent on some human, external connection. *But would this hurt my marriage?* I was asking this as quietly as I could and mostly to myself. I had requested Hank's permission to have a friendship with Oz and was tentatively updating and checking in with him. When Hank had crushes, I got the feeling he kept it under wraps and felt more entitled to it. It felt huge to challenge the box as a woman. I was guilt-ridden and felt responsible for maintaining Hank's manly image in our community.

But there was also an exhilaration starting to grow. A new thought of bucking the whole system and doing it my way, whatever way that would be, was evolving. I was just beginning to play with the possibilities of breaking the rules, and setting up new rules that worked for Hank and me and everyone involved. I was riding on a wave that had always served me—the openness to a new way of thinking—the ability to latch on to a great idea, and let it transform me. This, coupled with my attraction to Oz, started brewing a perfect storm of change.

I needed my world to expand so that it could contain more of me. In my current conundrum, one part of me was homebound with Hank. But I was foiled at home, holding back the part of me that yearned for more. Erotic energy is perhaps the most powerfully vital and unstoppable force of change. It has reordered nations, religions, and the world many times over. The erotic love that started growing on my walks with Oz would gather speed like an engine—and in the next two years it would become an unstoppable force that would reorder my life.

Chapter 6

Oz and I started taking walks together in October. It would be two years before the idea of opening my marriage was given to me. But it was the beginning of radical change. Timidly, I told Hank I had a crush on Oz. It felt liberating to negotiate having a friendship that was tinged with sexual attraction. Oz was affable and respectful to Hank. This contributed to Hank's acceptance of the situation.

As part of our work together, Oz hired me for three wellness coaching sessions. The sessions included learning how his workaholism was controlling his life and teaching him meditation. In an effort to interrupt his workaholism (which I defined as the neglect of his body and avoidance of his emotional world), I asked him to define love, to see if by his own definition he was loving himself. He defined love as "courage in the face of rejection," which revealed a whole new can of worms. I found him a fascinating subject to coach.

But in December, Oz took a prestigious job at a green tech energy start-up devoted to harnessing wind as a power source and canceled my services. I was hurt but partially relieved, since our friendship felt lopsided. After Oz ditched me, I got tough with myself. It was one thing to be a servile suck-up; it was quite another to be an *unappreciated* servile suck-up. After all, what did he bring to the table as a friend? I felt marginalized by his cancellation of our third wellness session. I decided to let the friendship fade away—sure he would never notice my absence.

But an odd thing happened. Oz courted my friendship. When I feigned busyness, saying the earliest I could walk with him was next month, Oz booked the walk, stating it was "ridiculously too far in the future." Then he added, "I believe there's this possibility of an awesome, everlasting friendship between us, and I want to nurture it as much as possible." He even dangled little teasers: "I can help you with all your technical computer problems," which was like offering sight to a blind man, since simple computer issues routinely daunted me. Two years earlier, I had produced and written a twenty-minute independent film—and I still hadn't figured out how to post it to the website I used to promote my acting and directing. Oz offered to do it for me, saying it would be "easy to do." It was an enticing offer, but I was wary.

We met up at Oz's house in late January on Martin Luther King Jr. Day. It turned out, given both our genuinely busy schedules, that a playdate with our boys was the only way to get time together. We had a blowout water fight with Merlin and Liam, which escalated from water guns to me hurling a bucket of water at Oz—over his newly varnished oak floors. After the water fight we sat down, and within a few minutes Oz confessed to one of the reasons he wanted to be friends.

"I want to be more like you. You have so much more space to play with in the physical, emotional, and spiritual realms."

Oz's admiration was unexpected. We talked for nearly an hour, and I opened up to him about my childhood and my daddy issues. The next day he sent me an e-mail:

> I'm in the particular place where (it seems) that I'm more angry at your dad than you are. Whenever we talk about it, I can't escape to my head, or say something caring, because I'm so angry.

I wrote back, thanking him profusely and expressing my affection.

Then the worm turned exactly in the way I had expected. Oz wrote me a three-page e-mail lecturing me about getting over my "childhood issues" by having "a conversation with your insecurities" and telling them to "shut up." Just as I was drawn in to him, I became equally repelled. I stopped e-mailing completely. During that week Oz sent three apologetic messages.

> I care about you…Please respond. It doesn't have to be a gargantuan screed about our respective places in the universe. Just reply "message received."

I finally crafted an epistle that basically said, "How about you attach my film to my website—to win me back?" I needed to stop fawning and demand respect.

The next day, Oz e-mailed a link to my website. A new page had been added. I pressed the link and miraculously my film played. I knew this was no small feat, so I wrote an e-mail titled "In Gratitude." I printed out my e-mail and Oz's response, which Hank found lying next to my journal, where I'd left it like a sloppy teenage girl drunk on her first swig of scotch. Hank did not tell me he had read the entire exchange till the next day.

In retrospect, I think my actions at this time were a floundering attempt to make things better. I wasn't getting what I wanted from Oz. But the same could be said for Hank. I needed Hank to engage with me, not just sexually but in other areas of our life that needed tending to.

The night after reading the e-mail, Hank blew up while we were on our date and driving.

"Go off to your fucking precious Oz," he told me.

I got out of the car and walked for ten minutes, then called Hank on my cell phone.

"You're supposed to let me walk for five minutes, then cajole me back into the car!"

I wanted Hank to be more emotionally responsive and directly sort out what wasn't working with us. But this was typical Hank; if I hadn't called him he probably would have driven to Canada.

Back at home we talked at length.

Hank said, "You are spending all this time walking with and e-mailing Oz. I want you to put that into our marriage. I want you to end your friendship with Oz."

I agreed to do so. As much as Oz had hit home runs, I often felt like I was nursing him along, coaching Spock from the *Starship Enterprise* about what an emotion was, what it meant to be human. *Did I really need to work this hard in a friendship? Was this healthy for me?* I wanted more reciprocity in a friendship—it felt appropriate to move on.

The next day I sent an e-mail to Oz:

We have to bring this friendship to a close.

He responded:

Only by the giving of yourself through commitment do you end up with something bigger than yourself. You have done that with your family. Grace, if the situations were reversed, I'd do exactly the same thing.

And that was that. I was plunged into sadness, and a little shaky in my withdrawal from Oz, but I felt capable of toeing the line. It was time to adhere to the rules of the marriage box. Attractions outside of your marriage were bad—I felt shame for wanting more. Also, I knew our connection hadn't mattered that much to Oz—he was frozen emotionally. *Why rock the boat for what would ultimately be an unsatisfying friendship?*

At the time, if you'd have asked me to place a bet on who more easily could maintain this abstinence between Oz and me, I'd have put one hundred bills on Oz to win. If someone was going to screw it up, it would be me—I was the dark horse in the race to behave appropriately.

When Oz was my Pilates client, our ongoing debate about the relationship between mind and body, and specifically his emotions, was left a stalemate. Oz vehemently denied that he was repressing his feelings (a clear sign of someone repressing his feelings). But, over time, I'd begun to enjoy Oz's restrained manner. I let go of the notion that suppressing emotions was almost undoubtedly followed by a dramatic exploding of repressed feelings. It seemed that Oz was just self-contained. That's how I had begun to interpret his actions.

Until it all went down exactly like I had predicted.

The volcanic undoing of Oz's calm exterior started the night of the school auction. Before I had met Oz, the annual auction was a dull fundraiser that I was obligated to attend. But now that he was in my life (sort of), the auction was a thrilling, heart-pounding event I wouldn't miss for anything. Three months after Hank had asked me to end my friendship with Oz, this was my opportunity to "legally" get to see Oz, perhaps even talk to him! I trained for it like a prize-fighter, waking up at five in the morning four times a week to pump iron at a nearby gym.

An hour before the auction I felt like a kid on Christmas morning; I'd dreamed about it, longed for it, and now it was finally here. I had even shopped for a push-up bra for the occasion. I needed to find *the* push-up bra of push-up bras. *Pushing* up wasn't exactly the adjective I was looking for; I wanted a bra that served up my boobs like two giant ladles of hearty stew under a starving man's nose. I found what I was looking for at a small boutique near my home: padded, lacy, and wired to serve up those steaming breasts.

In front of my full-length mirror, I put on the bra and surveyed myself. I had a red velvet minidress that I had sewn and fitted perfectly to my conditioned curves. I put it on over the bra. I wanted to look utterly striking from across the room. Oz would see me like a comet in the night sky. He would be propelled toward me, magnetized to my beauty. We would talk for ten searing, profound minutes, and then he would replay those ten minutes over and over again in his mind like a near-perfect Walt Disney romance, and years later on his deathbed he'd mumble my name with longing.

I grabbed my large gold-sequined purse and stuffed a football into it. Several months prior, Oz actually used the phrase "throw like a girl" in my presence. I had challenged him to a duel of football throwing that never happened due to the demise of our friendship. I imagined us tossing the football in some private hallway, after he adjusted to the bright light of my stunning beauty.

But two hours into the auction, Oz was a no-show. I was gloomy; the room was packed with more than two hundred parents, and Oz wasn't one of them. I got another cosmopolitan and flashed my ladles at a hip music producer dad who I knew thought I was hot. We flirted for a few minutes. Then I moved around the tables covered with merchandise. The auction felt dead. I decided to fulfill my civic duty—buy something and leave. I walked over to my table of pals and put my hand on Hank's shoulder to convince him to exit as soon as possible. I waited patiently for a lull in the conversation. Good Lilith, all I wanted was to crawl into bed with a glass of Chardonnay and watch *Pride and Prejudice* for the eleventh time.

A long-winded parent started a speech on improving the soccer field. If I cut in then, I'd appear to be exactly what I was: a self-obsessed parent bored by the PTA agenda. Frustrated, I looked away, and there on the outside veranda was Oz. He stood surveying the country club campus, his body slouched in a way that exuded sadness. Then he walked off out of sight. I grabbed my gold-sequined bag and headed out the glass doors, scanning the twenty-foot-wide veranda. Oz stood about thirty feet away from me, staring off at the hills, his back to me. I walked toward him. I was soaring now, with each step my wingspan growing bigger. At the perfect moment Oz turned and saw me.

His expression almost stopped me in my tracks: his face went from gloomy to surprised and then to almost sublime gratitude. I walked the twenty feet between him and me. I suddenly felt self-conscious. I stopped in front of him. He was smiling, blatantly vulnerable, so relieved to see me. I felt suddenly vulnerable as well.

"Oz," I said smiling.

"Grace."

I unzipped my purse and pulled out the football.

"I believe when last we spoke you talked some football smack? The challenge is on, my good man."

Oz laughed. I tossed him the football; he tossed it back. He threw with a gracefully good technique, hurling the ball quickly, creating a tight spin. I commented on the artfulness of his throw and returned the ball—probably throwing like a girl, since I am one. But I noted with satisfaction that, although my aim was slightly off, the force of my throw put Oz off balance. After several minutes we stopped, a bit out of breath. Oz walked toward me holding the football by his side. We stood across from each other.

"Grace, you look so red and so unbelievably beautiful."

"Thank you," I mumbled.

Not once in the history of Oz had he commented on my looks. We gazed at each other—the warm spring breeze felt palpable between us. I wanted to reach out and embrace him, but I knew I wouldn't. I was surprised by the weight of his reaction at seeing me—it felt momentous, like a homecoming.

"You look sad," I said.

"Grace, I am in deep, druglike withdrawal from not walking with you. If a genie gave me one wish, I'd wish for a carbon-free energy solution for the planet. But if he gave me two wishes, my second wish would be to go on a walk again with you."

I was stunned. I had only dreamed that Oz had missed me. I'd achieved my goal past my wildest expectation. Here was the unforgettable deathbed memory. But I had not planned what to do next.

"I guess I should be getting back," I declared.

We'd been out on the balcony for at least twenty minutes. I didn't want Hank to come searching for me.

"Yes," Oz said, forever the gentleman.

"I am going to go find the bathroom," I said lamely.

"Could I walk you there?" Oz asked.

He walked me to the bathroom, and soon after Hank and I left the auction.

In the morning there was an e-mail from Oz inviting me to lunch. I called my East Coast best friend, Reenie. We'd been friends since I was ten years old and she had frequently acted as my "confessor" when I got into a tight jam. I described the situation in full.

She said, "You know how since 9/11 they have Code Orange and Code Green?"

"Yes," I said.

"And you never know what the colors really mean in terms of a terrorist attack?"

"Yes."

"Gracie, you are in Code Red—one wrong move and you two will land in bed."

I e-mailed Oz, declining his offer. I also gave him a referral to a therapist, since on the veranda he had said that he was considering therapy. It was clear that Oz was in somewhat of an emotional crisis. I had become his confidante and guide. I sensed that he was craving more emotional intimacy. Which baffled me—surely Susan was offering this kind of support? Instinctively I felt protective of him. I wanted to make sure that with me "going away" he had a support system of some kind. I was proud of myself for getting him help and not crossing the sexual line. Yet, I knew I could not handle being alone with Oz at a secluded lunch. A week of silence went by.

That Saturday afternoon I tested for my advanced Pilates certification. Afterward, I went to a friend's house and did celebratory tequila shots. I went to the bathroom to freshen up, texted Hank, and then, on a whim, standing at the bathroom mirror, checked my e-mail. That's when my eye caught sight of one from Oz.

Call me. I'm in Vancouver at a wedding in lockdown with my frat brothers. I miss you beyond words. And I have so much to say about therapy and more. Drunken courage in the face of rejection.

Oz

I felt a surge of energy soar up my spine. I looked at the time stamp of his e-mail: exactly twenty-four hours ago at eleven p.m. I wanted to write a stern e-mail in response, something like: *You are drunk and I am married. Good day, sir!* If I were starring in a Jane Austen novel that's what I would have done. Instead I drove like a maniac to the nearby Whole Foods parking lot. I pulled out my cell phone, noting with regret the low battery. I frantically dialed Oz's number, heard his phone ring, and then what sounded like someone manically fumbling to answer it. I pictured Oz's phone flipping through the air in some Vancouver hotel room. The call ended and I shook my head. The boy was flustered. I dialed again. He answered.

"I just got your e-mail. Talk to me."

The air crackled between us.

"Oh, Grace, I have so much to tell you. I saw Cathy."

"Cathy? Who's Cathy?" Had I been replaced so quickly?

"Cathy! The therapist you referred me to, I met with her. You are my muse. That's what I discovered, you are my muse! I told her about my family and she said, 'Given your upbringing of prizing the intellect and rejection of emotion, what gave you the courage to come and see me?' The answer came immediately: *because Grace said it would be okay.*"

Given how frightened I knew Oz was to be introspective, I was moved.

"So, I inspire you?"

"Yes."

We both paused. It felt almost eerie to be talking so openly.

Oz continued, "Before I met you, I thought the feminine was weak. I didn't see how spirituality could benefit me. But you are grounded and spiritual. You're feminine and strong. You opened me up to a whole new world. I was so depressed before I met you."

I was both flushed with pleasure and embarrassed to be adored like this—it couldn't be right. Somehow he was missing my glaring flaws.

"Do you judge me for fawning on you? Do you think I'm silly?" I asked.

"Do you think you're silly?" Oz replied.

I liked how he'd flipped the tables on me, answering a question with a question, making me take responsibility for my self-esteem.

"I can't help it, I just like who you are. I want you to know that," I said. Then my voice faded, I wanted him so badly. "Hey, do mind me calling you Oz?"

"My grandmother used to call me Oz."

"Your grandmother? That's very sexy."

Oz laughed softly, "I don't think of you like I did my grand-mother. When you call me Oz it gives me street cred. I've never had street cred."

"'Osborn' didn't give you street cred?"

"Surprisingly, no!"

We both laughed.

"Grace, if I could imagine my perfect woman, it would be you."

A tingle went through my body. I felt like I was holding my breath. If wild bandits had approached my car and demanded my cell phone at knifepoint, I would have bitten their digits off to knobby, fingerless hands. I knew enough to chalk up Oz's words to drunken grandeur from someone who needed therapy more than he needed me, but still—I was hooked. I wanted him in every possible way one person can long for another. As the window of my car steamed with my own breath, his presence felt almost tangible.

I breathed, "Tell me about your sexuality. I am so curious about it. You are so much the tamped-down librarian…what are you like in bed?"

I felt like an alcoholic after a period of abstinence. I watched myself unscrew the bottle of gin and down several gulps. Oz started to answer—but then, miraculously, the Universe intervened and my phone battery died. I sat staring at my cell for several moments, incredulous. Then I drove the three miles home—very slowly, awed by what had transpired.

I woke up in the morning shivering with fear. One false move and I'd blow it—*Code Red*. Oz had texted me another impassioned missive. I couldn't think of what to do. Things suddenly felt wildly out of control. I decided to tell Hank that I was failing at our agreement to end my friendship with Oz.

"I am trying to tell Oz to go away," I admitted to Hank, "and it's not working. We need to show a united front. Help me."

In spite of the fact that it would surely cause Oz to despise me, I showed Hank Oz's e-mail, in which Oz declared he absolutely "had to see" me as soon as possible and that we should "take our relationship slowly" until "we know exactly what we are doing." I asked Hank to write Oz.

I felt a bit lame enlisting Hank to talk to Oz. But after last night's phone call, I was afraid of what would happen if I didn't nip this in the bud.

And yet, what transpired was thrilling: a three-way, intelligent discourse on what was actually happening. Hank wrote Oz an e-mail that started out as a scolding: "I am the cold slap of reality that you most definitely need right now…" It was stern but filled with tough love—something you'd receive from an older brother. Hank was almost coaching Oz.

You already have everything in your life that you need to be happy. I know what it is like to raise a family, be a lover and a father and a son… It is not easy. I'm sorry it had to come to this, but you are not welcome in my life.

Oz wrote back about an hour later:

This is the most righteous e-mail I've ever received. I thank you for it from the bottom of my heart. You are very classy for not ascribing blame. But I would like to say that I am sorry for what I did. It really was my intention to navigate in a direction that would work for all. But obviously that can no longer happen.

He asked permission to send me one last e-mail, which consisted of one line:

Grace, I will treasure the memory of you always.

After the storm cleared, I felt a multitude of contradictory emotions. I felt pain at losing Oz, but at the same time I was amazed by the intelligent, conscious way we had all spoken to each other. In the typical Hollywood script, I would have been cast as the "bad woman," and one of my men would have punched out the other, then carried me away. I felt embarrassed by my wacko-ness, but I also felt really loved by Oz *and* Hank. They both saw my nuttiness and *still liked me.* Hank and I had come to a relationship impasse and respectfully discussed it—no one got cast as the bad guy. It felt landmark. Hank had compassion for Oz, and vice versa. They were not adversarial.

Hank and I had a honeymoon period.

He said, "If every five years you blow a tire, I am okay with it."

It never occurred to me to discuss with him why I blew a tire—it was understood that I had wounds from my childhood and that I was kind of screwy. But a seed had been planted in me. *Was I so screwy? Or was I onto something—perhaps a new way of loving each other that allowed for more of ourselves to emerge?* Maybe we needed to make new marriage agreements that satisfied my "neediness"—not just around sex but money and emotional responsiveness as well. In couple's therapy I had discussed these areas, but little had transformed.

My attraction to Oz was the unconscious driver for change. Thoughts of Oz lingered. I imagined him up in the hills—*What was he doing? What was he thinking? Was he in a similar state of longing for me?* Quite honestly, I never once stopped thinking of him.

A few weeks after the great storm, Oz wrote me a plaintive e-mail, offering to be a source of "unconditional love" in whatever form could work for both our families.

> My wish is that everybody—you, me, Hank, Susan—could explore this idea later, and I mean later in units of months and years... Perhaps we could find a way that this could work, and benefit everyone...
>
> Namaste,
>
> Oz

"I see the divine in you" had been my standard ending to our Pilates sessions. Both the sign-off and his words moved me deeply. It seemed Oz was launched on a path of seeking the divine in himself—our friendship had changed him. With great sadness, I told him we had to stop having contact. His wife needed his exclusive attention. I felt concerned about Susan. As a woman I empathized with her. Oz had told me that he'd confessed in vivid detail his deep attraction to me, that our friendship had been "like a symphony" and made him feel "more alive" than he had in years, which made me uncomfortable. It seemed hurtful. I didn't want to be in between them any longer.

I wanted Oz to go into the great wilderness of his being and sort out his psyche without my help. I worried that he was using me as a distraction and salve to stave off this work. I could see he was scared. But I hoped Oz would stay the course in therapy and create a safe passage for himself. I could not stay and be a sedative for his process.

In his e-mail, Oz also mentioned that he was attempting to put back together the rocky pieces of his marriage. I felt sad for him. Hank and I were doing great—if only I could get off the smack.

Several months after the storm was over, I wrote in my journal, "I am *still* obsessing about Oz." All my friends said it would fade. I believed them. But after another few months I wasn't so sure. After six months I began to think of my Oz obsession as living with a terminal disease—you just accept it and go on. But after a year, I began to wonder, *What will happen next?* I was in the wilderness of my spirit—I prayed for help.

I would occasionally see Oz at school and say hello. It had always surprised me that he chose this charter school over the one near his house, which had an excellent reputation. The elementary school closest to my house wasn't that great, so I was thrilled when Tallulah won the lottery. Whenever I would see Oz on campus, I was pure cool on the outside, but inside I felt like I had won the lottery too. Once, we lingered well after the school bell rang, trying to pack a lifetime into thirty minutes, exchanging wishes for each other and epiphanies about our lives that were secret code for our longing. Each brief encounter stirred me up and made my heart lurch when it was over. Then months would go by when I would succeed in being more diligent in avoiding him, determined to avoid the pain of the inevitable good-bye.

After all these months, I was still thinking of the voice mail Oz left me the night at the Whole Foods parking lot. After my cell phone died during his drunken confession, Oz called back and left a short monologue answering my query about his sexuality. The memory of this voice mail haunted me. I'd erased it the next morning panicked—Oz and I risked hurting our spouses and children if we acted on our attraction. I had to expunge the voice mail, and the attraction with it. But erasing it had the opposite effect of making it go away. It became otherworldly, his words living on in me like a dream.

"Grace, I've never met a woman who I wanted to talk to as much as I wanted to make love to. I want to spend hours in bed with you, talking and fucking, fucking and talking. We once spoke on our walks about first kisses—how they were frequently awkward. My first kisses with you—and I am not talking just about the kisses I'd place on your lips but first kisses everywhere—would not be awkward, they'd be inspired."

After a year of pondering Oz's voice mail, for some reason a couples therapy session I'd had with Hank nearly twenty years ago came to mind. I had been feeling slighted that I was the one who frequently initiated sex, and I wanted Hank to seek me out as well. Our older male therapist, trying to help us, consulted his supervisor, who suggested a theory. She proposed that Hank was deeply in love with me but treating me "like his adored and respected wife" in bed. At the time I thought it was silly. *That wasn't it.*

But from my current vantage point her theory held credibility. I thought about my porn habit, which I used regularly to satisfy my raging sex drive. Hank found the porn distasteful—*I was married to a feminist!* Hank fully understood the degradation of women. He was the antithesis of my stepfather, a violent brute who adored my mother sexually and beat her.

Then I remembered a time, years ago, when I came home early, surprising Hank, who I found shamefaced leaving the bathroom holding a Victoria's Secret catalog. Sometimes I would sense late at night, when I rolled over in bed half awake, that Hank was masturbating in bed beside me. *Why couldn't he reach for me?* Was that female supervisor right? Were we both ambivalent about doing the nasty with someone we loved? Our relationship was tame and lovely. Oz's voice mail was lovely but also carnal. I couldn't stop thinking about it. It was the ghost in the room: lovely, ethereal, invisible, and ruling my psychic house.

I still believed the problem was me and my need for attention. My friend Freya was also struggling, with a narcissistic girlfriend she couldn't disengage from. Even though Freya was a brilliant child psychologist with tremendous emotional intelligence, she felt almost addicted to her girlfriend. Their relationship was like sipping a cocktail laced with nuclear radiation—the pretty glowing color drew you closer, the alcohol got you a little stoned; then you woke up in the morning with burned skin, your body filled with cancer cells multiplying by the second.

Freya and I decided to meet weekly doing co-counseling at her house in the heart of downtown Berkeley. After two months I was making progress, going for whole hours not thinking of Oz. Then one day, Tallulah, because of a series of unfortunate obstacles—lost shoes, a large snarl in her hair—was running late for school. I felt safe that I wouldn't bump into Oz, so I drove her to school. I was in my car, rounding the curve of a hill, moving at a solid good pace; we were now officially ten minutes late. The street was deserted like a ghost town. Then I got the tingle—a flash as if I were going into a wind tunnel where time was suspended—just as I came out of the curve. There was Oz walking alone. *What were the chances?*

As far as we were from each other, at least fifty feet, we both registered the other's presence. The air between us felt electrically charged. Our eyes locked. I felt myself lift my right hand off the steering wheel and wave, a very slight movement. Almost instantaneously, Oz did the same. Then the moment was gone and we were out of each other's sight.

I reported this event to Freya feeling cursed. I needed to purge all Oz thoughts again, start from scratch. I started reading about vision quests and fasts. So many of the great spiritual teachers had gone into the desert to cleanse and purge themselves and listen to the sweet voice of God. The magical number seemed to be forty days and forty nights.

Freya helped me map out forty days on my calendar. Unable to make a pilgrimage to the desert, I pledged to meditate an hour a day and record my random thoughts and beliefs about Oz. I also committed (yet again) to avoid the elementary school so as not to bump into Oz. A few weeks into my forty-day pledge I was talking to Freya about Hank and his pillow barricades, and my latest attempts to get close. I tripped over my words.

"I love Hank so much and most of our relationship is so satisfying."

As I was collecting my thoughts, Freya interjected, "Most of your relationship with Hank is unsatisfying?"

I was surprised by her question, since Freya was usually a meticulous listener.

"No, *satisfying*. My relationship with Hank is *so satisfying*."

"But you said it was unsatisfying."

"I did?"

"Yes."

I was suddenly frightened. If I said what was not working out loud, what would I have to do about it? I sat mute.

Freya smiled gently, "Why don't you talk about the ways that it's unsatisfying? You talk a lot about what works for you. What doesn't work?"

"Well, I—I know Hank loves me. His love has helped me so much." I stopped.

Hank was my home base. I had no other home, no family backup. He was my people. *What would I do if I lost him?* But I knew I had to step forward. This was the path of enlightenment that I had asked for. Like stepping across slippery ice, I started examining what was not working. I felt fragile. I knew I could change me, but focusing on Hank's changing felt abysmal.

Freya sat quietly, while I gathered my thoughts.

"Well...I don't feel desired. It's like Hank has no needs, he can outwait anyone. I want to make love with someone who really wants me." I paused, and then it hit me. I said to Freya, "I am going to keep getting these crazy crushes as long as I am with Hank. I am just not getting enough physical attention."

This realization was intimidating. I'd hidden it from myself for a long time. When I met Hank more than twenty years ago, we had been perfectly aligned and focused on healing together. But for the past decade I had been asking for Hank to join me in a rebirth of our sexual connection—and he was turning me down. My whole body felt heavy with the weight of what I was unearthing. My marriage had worked for a long time, but my needs had changed.

It was clear that Hank loved me and I loved him back, but it was also clear that a part of me would continue digging and clawing to find an underground well that would quench my thirst. This was the part of me that I had labeled as having "daddy issues." Maybe that had been true twenty years ago, when I had been wounded and impulsive. But perhaps now what I needed was a different kind of connection with my primary partner. This information was so frightening that I had no idea what to do. So I put it aside and asked again to be guided.

A few weeks later, Hank, the kids, and I went back east for Passover with Hank's family. We were close to where both Oz and I were raised, just a town away from each other. I felt Oz's presence with me during the trip. I started to feel a "quickening." This is the magical term associated with the first flutter kicks of your baby in the womb. Even though nothing had visibly changed, I felt that something was brewing. I secretly hoped it had to do with Oz. It had been months since I'd last seen him. I felt a premonition about him—like an impending birth.

The day after arriving home, as I got into my car and started the engine, I saw a man across the street wearing an odd-looking safari pith helmet. I noticed him because of the hat and the huge eighteen-wheel truck that came to a halt in front of him, forcing several cars to stop too, like the Red Seas parting as he crossed the street. He got closer. I realized with a start that it was Oz. Reflexively, I rolled down my window to say hello. But he walked past my car completely ignoring me.

What? *He didn't say hi?* I was devastated. I knew I was being silly—I had asked him to leave me alone. But how could he pass up a chance hello on the street? Even though these were the moments I agonized over with Freya, they kept me going. I went to the bank and then got back into my car, vowing to find Oz and make him say hello. But it'd been ten minutes, and I had no idea where he was going. I drove down the main drag anyway, when I noticed the pith helmet.

Oz sat at an outdoor café. I parallel parked and walked the thirty feet to the outdoor table. He was reading with his back to me. I tapped his shoulder, and he looked up at me.

"Can I sit down?"

Oz nodded. I expected him to be startled but he seemed serene.

"You didn't say hi to me," I said after I'd sat down.

"What?"

"You walked by my car—you ignored me."

Oz looked at me quietly. There was a whole new energy about him, a relaxed warmth of someone who had spent time sitting with all his wiry, uncomfortable feelings and found his way into a better place.

"Whenever I see the Grace Mobile I look away and think of something else. I'm sorry. I noticed your car was gone for the past week; were you out of town?"

He noticed my car was gone. I told him about my trip back east. I wanted to tell him that I felt his presence all week long. We sat looking at each other. I noticed the book by his side.

"What are you reading?"

"It's a book on the amygdala, the part of the brain responsible for playing frightening scenes over and over again. The facilitator of my men's support group recommended it to me."

The waitress arrived with a plate of pasta, which she set down in front of Oz. We both stared at the oval-shaped bowl.

"Are you looking at my carbohydrates?" he asked sheepishly.

I smiled. I felt so expansive sitting across from Oz, like I was touching all the stars in the galaxy. We told each other stories, asked questions about things we'd wanted to share for over a year. The last time I'd seen him we'd just nodded hello. The time before that it was just as brief. I was reminded again of the longevity of the attraction. Two years ago I had carried around a list with all of Oz's shortcomings and screw-ups. I would read it when I saw him at school, or in the street, or when I missed him. It was a brain-washing technique, like aversion therapy for homosexuals. And like aversion therapy, it never worked. A few months ago I had thrown the list away; I came to the conclusion that my feelings for Oz might be bad or immature, but I couldn't help it. He moved me and that wasn't going to change.

We stopped talking. I racked my brain to remember things I wanted to ask or tell Oz. I cursed myself for not writing down my questions; it felt urgent to pack it all in. Oz, by contrast, was sitting quietly, gazing at me.

"It's amazing," I said, "whenever I think about you intently I run into you."

"That isn't very scientific," he smiled. "Because I rarely run into you and, yet, I think about you all the time."

Oz thought about me all the time?! The news felt like salvation. Tears formed in my eyes—I ordered myself to get a grip.

"Grace, I want to tell you something."

"Yes?"

Oz paused, his words were measured. "I love you unconditionally. I know you haven't had much of that in your life. I love you completely and that isn't going to change. I can't see you and I shouldn't be talking to you now, but I want you to know how much I love you. Sometimes when I think about you, I am so filled with love.

I just hope you can sense it, grasp it, and hang on to it. I hope it makes you feel safer in the world, less insufficient."

I then understood what the Christians must feel like when they made pilgrimages to the sacred waters to heal themselves, when they soaked in those pools, the gratitude and redemption that must have flowed through them. I was crying now at the sidewalk café table. A mother I knew from Tallulah's school jogged by, her eyes looking startled when she saw me. This wasn't good. I looked back at Oz. It was striking how at ease he seemed, his eyes wide open, his gaze unerring. I couldn't think of anything to say, so we just kept looking at each other, and it occurred to me how potent that was, more so than any words we could say to each other.

It had to end. We both knew we needed to say good-bye. I stood up. I asked him if I could give him a farewell hug.

"No, I promised Susan I would never touch you."

I nodded. I respected that immensely. He was such a good person.

"Reentry is going to be hard," I said.

I dreaded what was coming. We had talked about this before. After brief contact, it took momentum to jump back into normal life.

Oz smiled gently but said nothing. We nodded the briefest of namaste head bows.

I walked the dead man walking to my car. I turned the key in the ignition and drove past Oz. I waved at him, and he waved back. I came to a stop light feeling the weight in my chest, when suddenly the undeniable realization poured over me—*I love Oz. I love him unconditionally too.* This love had been growing steadily even though I tried to kill it so many times.

I want Oz. I want Oz. I wanted all of him—as a lover, a companion, a friend. It was the first time I felt absolute certainty about it. I felt the quickening again; a rebirth was happening. Before this meeting I didn't trust my feelings for Oz, but seeing his perseverance, the positive growth he'd achieved—I knew he was a landsman of sorts. *Our love was a good love.*

I went home and called Reenie. She warned me that I was in a Code Red again. I called my friend Lila, an artist and confidante in my Oz odyssey. She reassured me that Oz would "not save my life or change it significantly. It doesn't matter who you are married to; work on your own issues." This should have been a revelation. *Yet… the ringing chant in my heart: I want Oz. I want Oz.*

I felt like I was hatching out of an egg and everyone was advising me to get back in the fetal curl and reassemble the eggshells. Something had irrevocably changed. For so long I had seen my attraction to Oz as a symptom of my wounds. My brain and all my friends agreed. But I could feel my heart and my spirit breaking out of the shell. There was a better way, and although I could not figure it out, I was sure some being, some spirit, knew the way through.

I had a great love with Hank. Why should I lose that? There had to be a way to preserve the love and the family we had created. Cracking our life apart with a divorce was not the answer. I was ter-rified to lose the stability, the daily connection to my kids and domestic life. I had fought too hard to create this life—I refused to give it up.

But I could not turn away from the magnitude of my love for Oz any longer, my heart and my body yearned for him; there was an intelligence in my yearning that I had denied—until now. Now my love for Oz was bursting forth and demanding that this new life happen. Somehow I had to have both men, my family, my children, love, great sex. How could I crack open my life and merge both worlds?

This was a substantial love and yes—an inconvenient love. I needed to be a family person, but I also needed to become more of who I was. I needed to express my sexuality with a lover who desired me as much as I desired him. Seeing Oz, in all his magnificence, having continued on his journey of healing and wholeness, without me but inspired by me, I could feel there was a journey waiting for us to take together. Before, I had seen this as a negative impulse to stray; I now saw it as a wondrous gift. For years, even before Oz, I had been putting out a call. Oz had answered it. He had proved himself an exceptional being by continuing his inner evolution without me. I felt afraid of this urge to have more, but I knew that if I didn't take the journey something precious would be aborted and gone forever.

I called Freya—I needed a witness. She listened quietly. My kids came home, and I snuck out onto my balcony that overlooked the street. I described the scene at the café.

Freya said slowly, "You are talking about Oz in a new way. I've never heard you use this kind of language or tone."

Yes! We were in a new place! Freya could see it too. At just that moment Oz drove by in his silver Fiat. My whole body jerked. *I want Oz!*

In the years during my Oz odyssey I had called on infinite spirits and collective intelligence for guidance. Standing on the balcony holding my cell phone with all the airwaves floating around me, I felt an almost visceral connection to an invisible network of thoughts and intelligence. I couldn't think of any one Goddess or spirit to call on. *But I felt an immediate urgency—a need for an answer now.* So, I did what witches occasionally do in a serious moment of need. It's sort of like ringing the emergency alarm bell, tearing the protective coating off and breaking through the glass. *I needed a sign! I needed a miracle NOW!* It was dicey to be this demanding with the Universe. It could show a lack of faith, like a petulant child.

I WANT TO BE LOVERS WITH OZ! SEND HELP IMMEDIATELY!

Give me a new alternative. I don't want to hurt Hank or my children, I won't lie or hide or get a divorce, but Goddess, I WANT OZ!

I went inside and made dinner with Hank while the kids played nearby. After dinner I wrote the final check to pay for that year's witchy retreat. I put a stamp on the envelope, making it ready to send.

I waited for my return call.

Chapter 7

In our sessions with Lily, Hank expressed tremendous fear that we would lose each other. I wanted to help him, to wipe away all his fears, because I was in such a different place. In my research on open marriage, I had stumbled on a word coined by a poly commune in the 1970s: *compersion*. Basically it is the state in which a person feels joy when his or her partner has pleasure with a lover. That is how I felt at the thought of Hank taking a lover. It seemed that we had stagnated in terms of helping each other out sexually. But it was clear to me that pleasure was the antithesis of trauma. Our intention had always been to heal from trauma together. I was clear we both needed more ecstasy, *even if the source would come from other people.* But to my mind, we could still retain all the good connection we had together.

All our friends were concerned. People were alarmed by what they felt was a risky venture. But when I look back at this time, what I recognize is that I needed a transformation, and I was willing to face the consequences. I wasn't interested in thinking about a downside—I needed energy to manifest a new life. When my friends warned, "You're playing with fire," it didn't stop me; it didn't even slow me down. I *was* the fire—a fire of enthusiasm to get laid. For years I'd been tempted by beautiful men who'd slink up to me at the gym, open their lovely mouths, and say, "I know you are married but if there's something your husband isn't giving you, let me give it to you."

Something my husband isn't giving me? Are you kidding me? While Hank was building pillow barricades, I was slipping my fingers into my wet slit, fantasizing about the boys at the gym, muscles bustling upon more muscles, pumping iron rhythmically, their bodies sheathed in a light film of sweat, their sweet young mouths saying over and over, "Let me give it to you, let me give it to you, let me give it to you…"

I was Christ in the desert being tempted by the devil nearly every day. I stayed in shape, I was attractive, I bought lingerie—*and for what?* Try as I might, no Tantric workshop, no therapist's office got me over the pillow barricade. In my twenties I was in a small coven of witches. One of my coven sisters used to say, "You know what I like in a man? I like a man who nearly breaks his legs running to get into bed with me." Me too, sister. I wanted to have sex—legally and guilt-free with a man who was thrilled to touch me. My desire had the velocity of a fire hose drowning out all recriminations and warnings. Most people were trying to focus me on preserving what I had. But I had been doing that for years, working with what I had, and I still wasn't getting laid. *I need dick, people. Stop talking sense to me!*

I did love Hank. He was my compadre, my foundation, and the only man I'd ever wanted to reproduce with—but working this hard to get laid once a month was just plain unjust. I wanted to make love every day. I wanted to make love as a way to get closer, to meditate, to go to sleep, to wake up, to fight. I wanted sex to be a wild playground for fantasies and a path to heal my demons. But Hank and I were out of sync. I wanted more sex for so long that I was ready to burst at the idea that I could finally get what I wanted—elsewhere.

One of my polyamory books outlined a philosophy that inspired me. The book described couples in which one partner was into some sexual activity but the other spouse had no interest. The idea was that, with communication, clear boundaries, and agreements, a person could satisfy those needs with someone else, someone who wasn't building pillow barricades but fluffing the pillows and hollering for a girl to get her sweet ass into bed. Basically, why throw away a relationship that worked ninety percent of the time? Why throw away all your connection with your mate, your assets, and your family life because one or two things were not on the menu?

The idea that someone could take me away from Hank was a distant possibility. I believed it was possible for me to become lovers with a man I loved deeply—maybe Oz, or someone else—and remain bonded with Hank. I was hoping that Hank and my new lover could coexist. But I didn't dwell on these possibilities too long. It was like I had been starving and now was ready to gorge at a feast, and someone was warning me that I might get indigestion. *I don't care!* The multitude of possible concerns was just not my primary focus at this time. I would work it out later.

Opening my marriage to another lover was a great idea no one could talk me out of. Some of my friends had happy marriages but rarely had sex with their spouses. These same friends tried to convince me that sex was not that important. It's what my friend Lila said, adding, "You should focus on your marriage instead."

I understood that people like Lila had long-term, successful marriages that were relatively sexless—which was fine if both spouses were synced up in this area. But sexlessness wasn't a part of my value system—I wanted daily ecstasy—and I was focused on my marriage, which is why I knew I had to open it.

Maybe sexless cohabitation was working for Lila and her spouse; or maybe, like for me, it wasn't—maybe it all seemed okay on the surface while long-term resentment decayed its foundation. Sex drive could cause resentment as much as misalignment in any area— money, childrearing, division of work—but when it came to solving the problem of sex drive, many people were saying to me "just be happy—don't take a risk." Their message was "don't rock the boat— longevity at all costs." But I didn't want to be in a marriage where longevity was its sole purpose for existence. There seemed to be a cultural obsession with hitting the fifty-year golden anniversary. If everything was working and you hit fifty years—fantastic. But fifty years just to hit fifty years seemed pointless.

I was willing to take a risk to set up a marriage that worked on my terms. I needed to have sex. If Hank and I set up sexual relationships with lovers outside our marriage and stayed together happily for fifty years, then, by my definition of success, we were successfully married.

I didn't want to become one of those couples—married decades, barely talking, no sweetness left in their connection—yet determined to hit the golden anniversary. The thought of these couples scared me. I had failed to entice Hank into more sex—but I was still sweet on him. I was willing to be sexually satisfied elsewhere and have my primary relationship be mainly emotional. But if I didn't get some action, I would become half of one of those unhappy couples. I had a frightening image of myself: an old woman, maneuvering my walker down the sidewalk, making bitterly sarcastic quips, as Hank hobbled behind me, my adult children muttering quietly, "They should have divorced years ago." No thank you. Opening my marriage was worth the risk.

After several sessions with Lily, Hank was still stalled. So I told him, "You go first. Go out into the world and find a lover. I will do nothing but support you in this endeavor." I welcomed Hank getting in touch with his passion. I wanted to sell him on the idea that we could have each other *and* great sex—even if that meant great sex with other people. Giving him freedom to explore on his own, not worry about me hooking up with someone, would surely move his thinking forward. Eventually, I imagined us both with lovers, going out on a date night separately once a week. I did not think this would disrupt our family life and that, in fact, our kids would never have to know. I imagined us with happy lovers on the side. It just did not occur to me how complex it would be—but even if it had, I would have walked the same path. I needed a change.

One day I went into Hank's office. He was typing away, his fingers energized on the keys, his face glowing with the light from his computer screen. "What's going on?" I asked. He sheepishly looked up.

Hank—the little slut—was carrying on a flirtation with an old girl-friend he'd connected with on Facebook. I peered over his shoulder at her Facebook page. I remembered Penny. Hank showed me her picture leaning against her large black stallion. She lived on a small ranch in Oregon. Hank said she was like a nervous schoolgirl.

"She doesn't want me to visit because she's put on twenty pounds."

I pulled up a stool next to Hank.

"Tell her it doesn't matter in the least, that you love extra padding."

Hank tilted his head, "So much flattery?"

"Women love flattery."

A week later Hank was on a plane to Oregon. Penny mentioned that she and her former boyfriend were no longer lovers but still "shared the ranch" due to financial entanglements. I couldn't resist sending Hank texts every few hours, "What's happening now?" I was home making pasta and playing cards with the kids but getting a vicarious thrill from Hank's escapades.

Apparently, Hank and Penny made out most of the night. Penny was fascinated with me and my ability to share Hank. I was fascinated by me too. It was like discovering you were a saint. And while other saints had the ability to take ecstatic flight, talk to animals, subsist without food or water for months, you had the ability to be really happy for your husband when he got laid. I never would have guessed it in myself. I could be righteously petty, an obnoxious driver leaning on the horn when someone hesitated even a nanosecond before making a turn. *Who knew I was the queen of compersion?*

The next morning Hank met Penny's boyfriend, Roger. When Penny was grooming her favorite horse, Sassy Boy, Roger appeared. He briefly shook Hank's hand. But when Hank returned home he received a crude e-mail from Penny's boyfriend threatening to "get on a plane" and "beat the living shit" out of Hank. We were morti-fied and *scared*. The e-mails kept coming, with escalating obscene threats interspersed by e-mails from Penny reassuring Hank that Roger would cool down and asking when they could see each other again. Hank sent an e-mail to Roger saying he would "never contact Penny again" and "never set foot on their ranch" or, for that matter, anywhere near Oregon. The e-mails stopped.

We were shaken. I ran this by my new poly friend Alex, whom I'd met through Lily. He had become my resource for poly advice. He and his wife, Chloe, had been doing poly for more than ten years. Alex said this kind of drama happened when you were new to poly and not to worry, we'd get the hang of it. He recommended surrounding ourselves with poly friends. He and Chloe were a part of a large poly community.

On our first walk together, Alex told me that Chloe was his "submissive" and any of their group of buddies could call up and ask Alex if he could have sex with her. I was both appalled and turned on. Alex described a weekend vacation that he, Chloe, and several of their group took in the country. He and Chloe created a "scene" in which Chloe was blindfolded, tied to the ground, and then fucked by twenty of their closest friends.

Alex went on to describe their community of poly pals. They watched football games together at their loft, and if someone wanted to get a blow job, chase a playmate around the couch, or act out some fantasy—have at it. There were also a bunch of daddies in the group but not the PTA kind: men who loved to both nurture and sexually dominate their women. My feminist brain had short-circuited and I was wet. What a conclusion to my daddy issues—*get a guy who actually wants to play daddy*. I loved the sex-positive attitude; no one was going to shame me in this crowd for wanting more sex and attention. Finally sex was on the table—guilt-free.

Some of Alex's pals were into plushophilia: they liked to dress up as stuffed animals and have sex. This pushed my limit of what was feasibly a turn on. I was with him on the daddies, even on sharing Chloe with his pals, but sex with people dressed as stuffed animals?

But I liked Alex. He had told me that when my waiting period was over with Hank, he'd be interested in dating me. I was flattered— sort of. I mean, who would Alex not date? He had about twenty lovers in circulation. I couldn't imagine who'd be turned down: someone with a worn Winnie the Pooh costume? I also noticed that Alex had not asked me much about myself. Still I did not judge him or his pals. I liked these sexual outliers; I considered them sex artists. This was their creativity, and they were devoted to it. But it was not quite my thing. I wanted a deeper connection.

The greatest thing about a poly counselor was her referrals. A few weeks after the Penny debacle, Lily told us about a poly meet and greet. It was quite close to our home, which astonished me. Just blocks away existed a sexy parallel world in which throngs of suburbanites were doing the wild thing into the quiet, crescent-mooned night. Perhaps I was projecting my imagination onto the event. Lily was rather vague when she gave us the information, simply stating there was a poly party that met up once a month. Hank and I decided to go; we made an agreement that I would just be there as support. This would be a chance for Hank to possibly meet someone.

When we arrived at the small California bungalow, the front door was wide open. We walked in tentatively, finding ourselves in a large living room. The furniture was pushed aside; there were lots of pillows scattered around the floor. A queen-size bed sat in the middle of the living room, with gauzy see-through curtains surrounding it. We heard voices and made our way to a narrow shotgun kitchen.

Nancy, our hostess, introduced herself. She wore a madras skirt and flip-flops. We explained we were friends of Lily. Nancy smiled cordially as her boyfriend, Rome, entered the kitchen. His blue eyes worked me over quickly, and then just as swiftly he became the polite host offering drinks.

We got plastic cups of wine. I felt a prickly tingle move up my spine as I surveyed the room of about six other strangers. They were all youngsters. I glanced at Hank, who seemed to have developed a film of sweat across his brow. The term "middle-aged" floated into my head. How pathetic we must seem to the youngsters, opening our marriage midlife. We stood silently.

I started homing in on the conversations around me; the twentysomethings were talking about their temp jobs and landlords. I felt teleported back to my youth as a bike messenger and actress in Manhattan. *I can do this.* I internally willed myself to make conversation.

I moved over to a woman who was seated at the kitchen table. She wore large sparkling earrings. There was a smattering of unopened corn chip bags next to her on the table.

"I love your earrings," I said.

We started to chat. She was a yoga instructor. After a few minutes we realized we had both taught briefly at the same studio. I felt my cool factor rise exponentially. I wanted to get a megaphone and shout, *I teach PILATES!* A few more people showed up who, thankfully, looked older. A guy decidedly more mature shook my hand. I was confident he would understand the concept of equity, my measurement of adulthood. There was no one in the kitchen that looked responsible enough or burdened enough to have procreated, but, regardless, I started to enjoy the party, chatting up the small crowd around me. The kitchen began to feel packed.

I looked over at Hank occasionally. He and Nancy were still talking. There were drops of sweat sliding down his face. I made my way across the room. On closer inspection, Hank looked clammy. There were large sweat rings around his armpits.

Nancy said, "You can take your shirt off. *Really, it's okay!*"

Hank was in an awkward agony, an introvert wanting to crawl back to the safety of home. I saw him with fresh eyes; he really was a stay-at-home model—it made me feel tenderness for him.

Nancy smiled at Hank with empathy. I was sure that if he could hang in there, there would be a mercy fuck in it for him. I decided to let Hank fend for himself as opposed to making him more self-conscious by mopping his brow. I started mingling again. It was an interesting crowd. There was an openness and sexual freedom you might find at a gay pride parade. Everyone was aware that they were doing something counterculture, so they were candid and inclusive when I asked questions.

I approached a couple that looked young both in age and demeanor. She sat curled in his lap while he explained that they were on a time-out from poly. During the last party he'd started necking with some chick on the back deck and his girlfriend flipped out. She said very little, her big moony eyes glued on him.

"Now we are going very slowly, staying very connected," he said.

I nodded respectively and thanked them for sharing with me.

A new couple in their forties arrived, and I moved in on them like a homing pigeon. She straddled her man's knee, wearing a flapper girl dress and nibbling chips. He wore a loud paisley shirt and had a distinctly effeminate air. I told them I'd just opened my marriage, and they encouraged me to fire away with questions. I asked how long they'd been poly and what their agreements were. They explained to me that they only did ménage a trois. I asked who they slept with.

"Different men," the woman piped up.

I wanted to come back with a jocular "You're one lucky lady!" but I decided this was too forward.

"Are these mutual friends?"

"Sometimes," she replied, "but also men we meet at swinger parties."

I took it all in without judgment. I was fascinated by my research. Then my phone rang. I instantly knew it was Hank. It occurred to me I hadn't seen him for at least fifteen minutes and hoped he'd gotten lucky with Nancy. I moved to the hallway where it was quieter.

"Hey," said Hank. He sounded worn out.

"Where are you? Did you float down river?"

"I am peeling my shirt off in the car. *Can we go?*"

As I walked out the front door, Rome said to a petite blond woman who was also leaving, "I am so sorry we didn't get a chance to make out!"

I got into the car with Hank.

"Feeling a bit tense, dear?"

"Why would you think that?" Hank replied turning the key in the ignition.

I teased him without mercy as we drove to get a drink. But over martinis at César I described all my conversations.

"Wow," said Hank. "Now I feel like I missed an opportunity to learn about poly. You really talked to people. It just felt like a meat market to me."

We decided the sex-party scene was definitely not his thing. Hank took a long sip of his martini.

"What are we going to do?" I asked.

"I'll figure it out," Hank said, biting into his garlic olive.

The next day Hank put a profile on OkCupid. The whole online advertising-for-love thing turned him off. But he did it, reasoning that anything was better than sweating profusely at a meet and greet. A week later he got an e-mail from an artist in San Francisco named Valerie who designed apps for iPhones and did public art installations. They scheduled a phone call. That night I put the kids to bed and then crept downstairs. Hank was leaning against the dining room wall cradling his cell phone next to his ear, biting his lip and listening intently. I watched my husband with fascination. I knew his body signals. He was in the mating dance. I felt happy—maybe this woman would appreciate him like I did. He had a careful response to what seemed like a long-winded monologue on the other end. I quietly tiptoed away. Twenty minutes later he came upstairs.

"How did it go?"

"We are meeting at the museum tomorrow night," he said with wonder.

We both laughed, I clapped my hands.

"You're happy for me?"

"Yes!"

We had lost some of the magic that happens between lovers. Now it was back in some form, and it was exciting.

The next evening we stood in front of his closet picking out the perfect outfit. Who better than I to walk him through what clothes best showed off his assets? We decided on a black Calvin Klein T-shirt and a pair of gray trousers. The outfit said, *I am hot and I am trying—but not in a desperate kind of way.* He left for his date.

Four hours later he returned home in a trance. I asked for every detail. They had hit it off immediately. In the ticket line for the museum Hank had kissed her. The cold sweats at the sex party were gone. This was the man I fell in love with twenty-five years ago. Hank described every detail of the date. After their first kiss, Valerie had whispered, "We should go slow." He had moaned, "Do we have to?"

At the end of this description Hank asked again, "You're okay with this?"

I was more than okay. For years he had wanted me to go to museums, galleries, and other art-world activities that turned him on. I had wanted to go mountain biking, dancing, and have marathon sex sessions. Valerie sounded like the artsy girl he had been dreaming of. I was happy for him.

In his first week with Valerie, I twice rolled over to find Hank's side of the bed empty. I grabbed my cell phone and dialed, half expecting to hear his cell ring downstairs, but the house was quiet and a moment later his voice mail picked up. My stable, domestic Messiah had gone AWOL. Poly was like a young colt: wily and unpredictable. Hank arrived at six a.m. the next morning to get the kids off to school.

He asked to see Valerie again the next evening. I reminded Hank what he'd said about Chloe and Alex's two date nights a week with their lovers—"That's way too much time away from home." How things changed. Hank and I had agreed on one date night a week with Valerie, but I was okay upping it to two. Beyond the schedule of date nights, we did not have agreements about falling in love or what Hank could do sexually. We did agree on safe-sex precautions. At this point we had no idea how fast unpredictable situations could crop up, situations that were gray areas in terms of perceived agreements. But at the time I didn't feel we needed more agreements. I think we had come to take the stability in our marriage as such a given; it didn't occur to us that huge shifts could be happening that would require deeper contemplation to avoid future mishaps. But this felt like the right thing to do at the time. If we had tried to be perfectly aligned, reviewing every possibility, we probably would not have moved forward. And it was clear that we both knew, on some deeper level, that change in our relationship was needed.

The next night I came home to find the kids lying on their bellies, in front of the television, eating bowls of cereal. At this point the kids knew nothing of our poly life. When Hank went on his dates, we told them he was going out with friends. It was five thirty and Hank would usually be making a home-cooked meal.

"Where's Daddy?" I asked.

"He's taking a nap," said Tallulah.

I was furious. When Hank woke up I told him that he had to have enough energy to take care of his family. He agreed wholeheartedly, saying it would not happen again.

I joined a poly support group filled with people offering insights on how they did poly. Aurora, our group leader, wore caftans and had a lovely, voluptuous body.

She'd been poly all her life. During one meeting she described one of her happiest times: when she lived in Amsterdam and had four lovers, each fulfilling a separate need.

Her husband, John, was always there to greet me when I arrived early to the meetings. He'd open the door, smile confidently, then motion me inside with a welcoming gesture. Aurora would sweep downstairs, making a dramatic entrance. John would roll his eyes, chuckle, then make an equally dramatic bow to his fair lady as he headed to the kitchen to finish his dinner.

At my first meeting, Aurora had us do an exercise in which we identified our needs in a relationship. Aurora candidly declared that she loved attention and then went on to list the various ways her husband and lover responded to this need. I was floored by her unabashed self-acceptance, suddenly realizing that for years I'd been entombed in the belief that all my attention-getting antics were pathological, requiring years of therapy and/or pharmaceuticals.

Kitani, a man with the litheness of a cat, added that he also loved lots of attention. He purred next to me on the couch. His wife, Amelie, shook her head, laughing. "When I married Kitani, I told him, 'You better get a girlfriend too. Because there's no way I'll be able to give you that much attention!'"

Amelie was very matter-of-fact and completely without judgment. For more than ten years they'd been living together in a duplex, with his girlfriend in the adjacent flat.

Kitani sat beside me the whole meeting, purring and rubbing my thigh and glowing at me. I was the new poly girl on the block—and I was loving all the attention it got me.

Then Jessica offered shyly that she needed to feel "more empowered sexually." I listened transfixed. She and Manny were the last people I'd imagined finding at a poly meeting. He looked like a linebacker, muscular and squat with soft brown eyes, wearing a faded '49ers sweatshirt, his arm gently encircling Jessica, who had a perm that was giving me a gnarly '80s flashback. But I liked them. Jessica explained that she needed to experience her sexuality apart from Manny, whom she'd married fifteen years ago as a twenty-two-year-old virgin. Manny nodded quietly, then added that he'd played the field extensively before meeting Jessica, who he described as "the woman of my dreams." He wanted to support her happiness. Shockingly, the linebacker seemed to exhibit the feminist ideal that Jessica's sexuality did not belong to him. Furthermore, her evolution as a person was clearly important to him. Their devotion to each other was moving. In general, the whole group impressed me. I was struck by everyone's sex-positive attitude and their commitment to their relationships while being true to their needs.

At my second meeting I met a couple in their fifties. Marc was short and paunchy; Ianka had a thick Russian accent and only allowed her husband to have sex when she was there watching. I couldn't help but think this would be a buzzkill. Ianka was built like a small tank, and, although she was friendly, I couldn't help but imagine her whacking Marc's latest poly conquest over the head just as her husband climaxed. She attended the meetings with Marc weekly, saying she had "no interest" in other men but as long as she watched it "wasn't cheating." Mark and Ianka were looking for a woman to form a triad. They wanted to recruit Aurora but she wasn't interested. They'd been eyeing me ever since I'd walked through the door.

When I checked in, I gave the update on Hank and Valerie. Ianka made soft snickering noises when I described Hank returning home at six a.m.

"Feels like cheating to me," she said.

To me it wasn't cheating at all—I had agreed to the situation. But something felt off. I needed help defining what it was. Aurora homed in on my predicament. The poly creed stated that jealousy was an umbrella feeling that could mean anything from loneliness to anger.

"What do you need to feel good about Hank and Valerie?" Aurora asked.

I pondered her question. "I feel a bit betrayed. I am happy for Hank, but he's not taking care of business."

Aurora flipped back a strand of her ultra-chic bob.

"Do you feel territorial?"

That was exactly it. In the poly handbook there is the phrase "new relationship energy." Basically, it's when you get a new lover and lose your nut, and your first partner has to sit by and watch while you behave like a lovesick puppy. Hank was getting sloppy about taking care of his family. He was still showing up late and tired. I felt like a dog that needed to piss in all the corners, marking her turf. Aurora assured me this was a healthy instinct to protect my family. His new relationship was infringing on our family life. This was one of those unpredicted situations; we needed to revisit our agreements.

One night Hank, again, didn't arrive home at the agreed-upon time. The next morning, the kids and I returned home with groceries to find Hank sitting in the living room waiting for us. I sent Tallulah and Merlin upstairs and informed Hank that we were officially in crisis. He sat alert, as I outlined his transgressions.

After our official crisis (which later we joked about, since what would an *unofficial* crisis look like?), things started to fall into place. Hank started coming home earlier and got enough sleep to fulfill all his duties.

Two months after starting his relationship with Valerie, and six weeks after the "official" crisis, Hank and I sat down to talk.

"I am so thrilled you're happy with Valerie," I said.

We held hands, crying and gazing at each other. He looked at me with wonder.

"Thank you." Hank said. "When you start dating, I want to be as generous with you as you are with me."

"That's sweet."

"Poly feels so different than I imagined it would."

"Like what?" I asked.

"I just never thought I could talk to you about being sexual with other people." He paused. "I feel like a teenager. Valerie and I have such great sex—sometimes twice in one night."

"Really?" I knew they were having sex but—twice a night? I felt off balance.

He saw the look on my face. "Oh, that was too much. I'm sorry!"

"No, it's okay," I said genuinely.

But I felt a searing pain in my chest. Why was he sexual with Valerie and not with me? It had been months since we'd had sex. I was trying to create a situation in which we could have each other, remain an intact family, but have sexual relationships outside of our marriage. That was the way I saw us doing poly. But I felt ashamed that Hank and I rarely had sex. Weren't you supposed to still have sex with your spouse even when you added in a new lover? Was I doing poly *wrong*? Would I too be able to find a lover who'd break his legs running to leap into bed with me?

Hank was watching me closely. I smiled at him, then touched his hand.

"Really, I'm okay."

In those first months that Hank and Valerie were dating it wasn't often that I felt jealous. I did feel protective and sometimes territorial about our family, but I was mostly happy for Hank. I felt compersion—it gave me joy that Hank was experiencing eroticism again. It helped that I really liked Valerie. I met her one night when I was feeling kind of lousy, and was struck by how easy it was to talk to her. She had dropped by the house after the kids were asleep. She told me, "Well, you may feel lousy but you look great!" I'd just sewed myself a new dress to ease my mood and appreciated that she'd noticed it. Aside from the compliment, I could see she was genuinely reaching out to me, trying to preempt any jealousy or competition that would be expected from the situation.

That night we talked and laughed for over an hour—me, Hank, and Valerie. Almost immediately it felt like Valerie and I were on the same wavelength. We had the same intention: to lovingly share Hank.

After Hank had settled in with Valerie, I floated the idea of me starting to date. He tentatively gave me the green light, saying again he wanted "to be generous" with me but admitted that he was still feeling threatened.

I put up an OkCupid profile. I mainly perused other people's bios with fascination. I got some inquiries on my profile from various men, but when I flashed over to their picture, I recoiled with alarm and chanted quietly, *There is no way, no way I could have sex with him, no way.* Most of the men writing to me seemed jaded. One guy wrote:

> My wife left me after twenty-five years. She just couldn't take it anymore.

This is how you sell yourself? My Goddess, it was scary out there.

But one day my luck changed. I got a witty e-mail from Trevor. He seemed quite sexy and erudite. He had pictures of himself at the Burning Man festival at Black Rock Desert wearing dark aviator sunglasses and striking dramatic poses against the stark landscape. Quite frankly, this worried me. My hip factor had really slumped in the past decade since having kids. As Tallulah put it to a recent visitor, "My mom goes to bed at eight thirty."

"Nine o'clock!" I had said defensively.

How does one come back from that? I had a reputation to uphold as a wild thing. But who was I kidding? The last time I felt like a sleek fox dancing the night away was a good ten years ago.

I was impressed by how extensively Trevor had studied my profile. He knew my stance on flag burning, which I realized with dismay that I couldn't even remember. Have I mentioned the memory loss after age forty? Apparently I was against flag burning. Who knew I was such a square?

After a few e-mails Trevor asked me to dinner.

"Let's do it," I responded bravely.

We met at an Indian restaurant in downtown Berkeley. My first impression was that he didn't look like his mega-hip Burning Man photos. There was an uptight quality to him, which was surprising, because he had been poly for ten years. We sat across from each other drinking wine as I tried to assess if I was attracted to Trevor. Dating after years of marriage was confusing. It was as if you'd been banned from eating sweets and suddenly you were sampling pastries, but you honestly couldn't tell if you liked what you tasted. We had a bad moment about twenty minutes into the date when I told him I'd lied about my age. He looked shocked.

"Why did you lie about your age?" he asked solemnly.

"Well, I feel much younger than I am…" my voice trailed off.

He looked offended. I felt off balance. Was it such a crime? The truth was, I didn't feel that I looked forty-six. I worked out. I looked about—*this is where things get warped*—I wanted to say *twenty-nine*, because there were days I felt that spry and sexy. But I'd done enough therapy to know this was from the part of my brain that housed the sisters of illusion and grandeur. So in my profile I added nine years to my *felt* age and broadcasted it as thirty-eight.

Also, I noticed I had mutual chemistry with men who were younger by about six years. Oz was nine years younger. I explained to Trevor that I had wanted to pick from someone in that age range. *I meant no harm.* He nodded. He seemed so serious. After an hour, I asked if he wanted to get a drink after dinner. I confidently put my arm into his as we walked down the sidewalk. We had drinks at a long black marbled bar, which upped the flirtation machine. But twenty minutes later, Trevor abruptly said good night and didn't even offer to walk me to my car, which was a bit scary since I had parked on a dark street near a park. I felt like bruised fruit well past its sell date.

The next morning I received a crisp e-mail:

I felt no spark, I am assuming you didn't either.

Now I felt like moldy fruit.

Trevor went on to write that lying about my age was not a good decision.

Age is so much more than how you look. It's what stage of life you are in.

Thanks for informing me of that, you immature twerp.

You more than deliver on your claims in the looks department.

This slightly placated me.

Then he suggested I do what some other old chick did in her OkCupid profile:

Say you are thirty-eight so you are in the search pool with younger folk, but explain in the profile your real age and why you have chosen to state otherwise.

He ended the e-mail saying he was "moved" by Hank and I opening our marriage after "so many years together." Now I felt like I was in the geriatric ward with an IV in my arm. I sent a brief "thank you for the advice" and signed off before he paid me anymore insulting compliments.

"I'd feel so much better if I'd axed him!" I wailed to Hank, who was working to console me while he prepared to meet Valerie for lunch. I could see Hank felt empathy for me but was also comforted by the fact that my date was a failure. He reassured me that Trevor was a jerk and advised me to "let it go."

I was a bit stung by my first foray into dating. But although I was worried about finding someone I'd have any chemistry with, I still felt optimistic. *I would do it.* I would find a stellar man the likes of Oz.

At our last good-bye three months ago, Oz and I had briefly mentioned talking after six months. We had promised ourselves a check-in, to see if his wife would allow us contact of any capacity. But at the time we had hung up, I decided it was over. I would force myself to get on with it. Oz was not available. Part of moving on was finding a lover that I was enthused about. I was determined to find someone else who would make my heart go pitter-patter with the vigor that it had pulsed for Oz. I prepared to get back in the game.

Chapter 8

After my date with Trevor, I polished my profile, explaining I was actually forty-six but looked—*Goddess what's the truth? I now felt sixty-eight*—perhaps forty on a great day? (Yes, I used Trevor's advice—it was *good* advice to be more honest.) I also added that I seemed to have chemistry with younger men but didn't specify how much younger. I decided to put some pictures of my midsection in my profile to back up my claims. Several men had sent me shots of their abdominals—*if the boys could strut their stuff, why not me?* I spent an hour trying to get the perfect abdominal shot with my cell phone, then posted two shots. Game on.

Within twenty-four hours I checked OkCupid. I noticed an e-mail from an engineer in Silicon Valley who worked on gaming software. He was superhot and—*twenty-four...? Huh?* I knew immediately that it was a hoax. I pictured him and his frat boy pals concocting an e-mail to play a prank on the nice red-haired old lady. But the boy persisted with several more e-mails telling me I looked "like an angel." Now I knew he was deranged, nobody—*I mean nobody, not even my mother*—has ever referred to me as an angel.

Over the next four weeks I was deluged by e-mails from younger men. Some yahoo in the deep woods of Canada was enthralled when I responded to his near-illiterate screeds; another adorable submissive dude promised to clean my house if I'd have sex with him. This was an especially compelling offer, given my equal parts of horniness and laziness. I was getting stoned on the man-drug: boys in their twenties hitting on me. It was candyland. After a week I had sold my soul to the shallowest forms of life—posting several headless body shots of me in workout gear: a red halter top and tight cotton leggings. I also posted a few shots of me in a leopard bra. I was like one of those newly famous Hollywood starlets with a cocaine habit: stoned, high on attention, and getting dumber by the second.

But after a few e-mail exchanges with these little twentysomething man-hos, I began to feel like a middle-aged man who leaves his wife for a youthful Playboy bunny and then realizes—*there's nothing to talk about*. Put simply, there was an appalling lack of life experience.

I missed Oz. Although all the attention was flattering, Oz was the standard. What would it be like to be lovers with Oz? After another week of sexy e-mails from twentysomethings, I did several searches on OkCupid looking for a poly guy with soul. This was challenging. Many poly guys seemed like they just wanted a steady flow of new ass in their life. I understood this modus operandi had a place in the poly community for both male and female poly players. It's just that I didn't want to be the rotating flavor of the month. I wanted longevity and an intellectual connection. I didn't want the poly man-ho, I wanted the poly prince: a man who would woo me and talk to me, and who was interested in all of me.

After an hour, I found a guy in San Francisco named Tom. I reread his profile several times and perused his ab shot. He was forty and looked like a young Willem Dafoe with sexy, soulful eyes. I hesitated. There was something just *a little slimy* behind the soulful eyes. But I had to jump in. I wanted to find someone that would erase the longing for Oz. I crafted a short e-mail, per the requirements in his profile: "Please write if you are fun and sexy and nice." I was praying he had some depth beyond his shallow requirements. I wrote:

I would say I am fun and sexy and nice. I am okay with poly since I am doing it as well.

That's pretty much all I wrote. What can I say? The guy had a low bar to jump over.

He wrote back almost immediately:

How have I missed you on OkCupid until now? I love that you are tall and fit and very, very red.

He had been married for fourteen years. He and his wife had opened their relationship a year ago. "We are happier than ever," he wrote, and then invited me to have a drink. I liked the enthusiasm. I needed enthusiasm after my disaster date with the square poly guy. We exchanged e-mails about poly and our marriages. He sent me a link to an article titled "The New Wave of Poly" that touted its feminist roots. It had been his wife's idea to open their marriage. He supported her sexual explorations. I booked the date. He suggested a bar with plenty of dark corners: Cyclops Cave in Berkeley.

We planned to meet at four o'clock on a Thursday afternoon. A few hours before my date I nervously put on my dating uniform—clingy red Michael Stars top, Paige denim miniskirt, black tights, and leather boots with three-inch go-go dancer heels—but I didn't feel entirely buoyant. I was afraid I'd have no chemistry with Tom.

I liked his e-mails, but I wasn't confident—you never knew who you're dealing with till it's live action. I was realizing it would be a challenge to find someone that truly excited me—on all levels. My worst fear was that we'd meet up and it would be flat, like with the uptight poly guy. I surveyed myself in the mirror. The miniskirt and boots made my legs look extra long. Tom's profile said he was six-foot-four, so I felt comfortable with the boots. I turned to survey my ass in the full-length mirror. *Does this outfit work for me?* Dating had lost its glossy fun.

I went downstairs.

"Do I look all right?" I asked Hank.

He looked up from his drafting table and said, "You look fantastic."

I needed the bolstering. Then perfunctorily I asked him, "Is my breath okay?"

I breathed on him. He flinched slightly.

"What?" I said alarmed.

Hank looked uncomfortable. Now I was really nervous.

"It's just—your breath is acidic."

"What?"

I was panicked. I had bad breath? The person with bad breath is always the last to know.

"You tend to get bad breath around your period."

"What?" I sounded like a parrot.

"You get this really acidic breath right before you menstruate."

"What?" *I have got to come up with a new word!*

Now I was really freaked. I ran to brush my teeth and gargle with hydrogen peroxide. It was thirty minutes before my date. At this point I'd have gargled with Drano if we had some. I grabbed some licorice lozenges from the cabinet. They were left over from when Hank had GERD. I remembered that they had neutralized acid.

"Jesus, how long have I had bad breath?"

"About since Merlin was born."

"What?!" It had now become a verbal tic. "Merlin is five years old! Why didn't you tell me?!"

Hank looked pained. He was trying to backtrack.

"Is this why you don't have sex with me?"

Hank was silent.

"I've had bad breath for the last five years and you didn't tell me!"

"I'm sorry!"

Looping thoughts circled my brain. *Why couldn't you have worked with me on our sex life? Why are you telling me this now—thirty minutes before a date?* My thoughts were interrupted by urgent Googling of bad-breath remedies. For the next five minutes I brushed, gargled, and ate a small mountain of mints. Then I breathed on Hank again.

"Better," he said, but he looked a bit scared.

It was not the one-hundred-percent endorsement I was looking for, but it would have to do. *Great.* I was heading out on a date with one of the rare guys I'd been excited to meet on OkCupid and I had just discovered I was one of those hygienically challenged people who cause you to lean back when they exhale in your direction. *Fantastic.* My confidence was shot.

I got into my SUV feeling like a real glamour girl. I aggressively chewed handfuls of breath mints as I drove. I arrived five minutes early and parked near Cyclops Cave. I was walking down the sidewalk when I saw a man two blocks off, heading my way. I knew immediately it was Tom. He had a relaxed, loping stride and was very tall. My brother had coached me with Internet dating wisdom: "Don't overjudge someone by a bad profile picture, have a mandatory call to prescreen for crazies, and when you meet someone in person—you'll know in the first thirty seconds whether it's a go."

I felt a tingling as Tom approached—my brother's wisdom was apparent. Tom had an easy gaze; his glowing brown eyes instantly found mine. We introduced ourselves. He told me he had to get money from the ATM. We walked the block to the bank. As he pulled a few twenties from the machine he made a joke about me not seeing his "pathetic bank balance." We giggled then started talking about money, kids, parenthood, his job as a veterinarian's assistant. Within five minutes I was sure that if he could survive that acidic first kiss, game on!

At the bar we exchanged stories. It turned out his wife almost left him.

"It was divorce or open our marriage," he confided. "I figured I didn't have much to lose."

We talked some more, then he asked me to move closer. He leaned in and I knew what was coming. I prayed that my mints and licorice lozenges had worked their magic. He deeply kissed me and then rubbed my upper thigh. He looked happy. *This is workable*, I thought. His kisses were nice… Then Oz passed through my mind. There had been a two-year buildup to a kiss that never happened. I realized quickly that I'd have to change my expectations. How could someone I just met an hour ago compare to the deep friendship I'd developed with Oz? We'd had more than twenty walks and nearly a hundred e-mails. I had to lower my expectations.

Later that night, Tom texted me during my poly support group. I was listening to the riveting news that Jessica was dating a guy named Samson. At first, Manny felt almost devastated, but he rallied and met Jessica and Samson at a sports bar, where they all had a beer together! Then Manny and Samson played a game of pickup basketball! We were all misty eyed at the news. I discreetly went to the bathroom to read Tom's message. I loved texting—it felt like passing notes in school. Tom was already rearranging his schedule to see me sooner. *Me likey.* Somebody wanted to have sex with me and was talking sweet to get it! I thought of Hank and all the years I brushed up against him in bed, infiltrating his pillow barricade, gently rubbing my pelvis against his butt, to hear him say, "Not tonight." Not even a "dear," as in "Not tonight, dear." Once I'd even replied, "If you are going to say no can you at least do it nicely?"

As happy as I was to be courted, I was worried Tom was going to try hustling me into bed. Oz had been willing to sacrifice any physical relationship to have the pleasure of my conversation—*my words* moved him. I wanted that experience again. I wanted a man who was so into me he would wait to get *into* me. I texted Tom explaining that I just wanted to "make out for a few dates, and take it slow." He replied that that was "fine"; although he was "excited to be physical" he would honor my wishes.

He also explained more of who he was: "in a relationship, my tendency is to be pretty attentive." He said he liked "talking and checking in," but he didn't want me to feel "encroached." He wrote:

> I am not a stalker. I just like to interact with the people who are close to me… I realize that for some people, this type of constant attention can be overwhelming.

"Constant attention" is overwhelming? This guy had no idea who he was dealing with. *I wear out stalkers.* I e-mailed back.

Stalk away! Stalker is my type.

I liked this dude.

The following night he called, and we planned a date in San Francisco. As we were chatting, he brought up Addison, the other chick he was dating. He had mentioned her at Cyclops Cave. When he said her name what immediately popped into my head was *That girl is so history once you taste my world-class pussy.* Then I realized that was hardly the poly creed. I had to play by the poly rules and pretend to approve of his slutting around.

The evening of our date I raced into the city early. I wanted to be prepared for any impromptu make-out sessions. There was a great lingerie shop in the Haight District that sold 1950s corsets with a garter belt to attach the stockings. Meeting in the Mission District with "no bed" was a fashion challenge. As I saw it, the difficulty about fooling around in a car or in the streets was the possibility of arrest or worse still: the rumpled look after making out. I accepted this fashion challenge with enthusiasm.

I stepped inside the curtain-draped dressing room and quickly squirmed into the form-fitting corset. I gazed at myself in the dressing room mirror. It was exactly the look I was going for. The black crotchless corset hugged my curves; I adjusted the silk stockings and struck a Betty Boop pose. This was an easy-access outfit. I imagined Tom guiding me into a dark alley, lifting up my dress, and penetrating me with his fingers, as I leaned back, wet and ready—*a fulfilled yet intact fashion icon.*

When I entered the restaurant in a clingy black wrap dress that covered my corset and stockings, Tom jumped up from the table, nearly knocking over the salt and pepper. I could tell he was one of those skinny guys in high school who never got laid, which made him eternally grateful to any woman willing to spread her legs for him. Tom pulled out my chair and I sat down at the small table in the crowded tapas bar. We chatted. He was easy to talk to. We drank sangria. After an hour, he leaned in.

"I feel like you are giving me mixed messages."

"How is that?" I sounded a bit smug, like I had just been coronated The Queen of Pussy. *Here I sit omnipotently perched on the desired pussy.*

"Well, you said you wanted to wait to have sex, but then you made that comment tonight about our hotel budget."

Tom was budget conscious. I got the feeling he didn't want to blow money unless there was guaranteed sex. My brain started to float to thoughts of Oz. My conversations with him were so textured. He never missed a beat, and he would pick up on all my complexities.

"I just meant that we could make out in a hotel. But I know you don't want to blow our budget on a make-out session."

Tom nodded. His eyes glowed.

"I want to ravish you."

Ravish? Did he just say "ravish"? This was only the second time I'd heard a man use that word. Oz had said that to me in our last ill-fated conversation four months ago. Oz. Why did he always have to pop into my mind at these moments? Why was I continuing to compare every other man to him? Here I was with someone eager to fuck my brains out and all I could think of was the last time Oz and I had said good-bye. After our chance meeting at the gas station, when I'd told him I was opening my marriage, Oz took a month of contemplation then decided, "I've got to try again to make it work with Susan."

This was my odyssey with Oz, chance meetings where we urgently tried to pack a lifetime into a brief conversation. At the end of that abysmal call Oz said, "We've said good-bye so many times we should be getting good at it." We both laughed and then wept. I felt like someone was physically removing my heart, a surgeon snipping through my arteries, my life's blood draining away.

"You're doing the right thing," I said to him, wiping away my tears, "It's the right thing to fight for your marriage."

I admired Oz. He was taking the high road. But the honorable decisions he made *took him away from me.* It was a miserable predicament. At the same time I wanted him to go. *Just go! Go! Let me salvage the rest of my bleeding heart!*

In that moment I was turned upside down with pure vulnerability.

I stammered, "But if I were single and you were single you wouldn't go away? You are attracted to me—right?"

Even over the phone I could hear Oz take a deep breath. His voice was so male, such a deep timbre.

"Grace, if you were single and I were single, I would ravish and ravish and ravish and ravish you. I'd never stop ravishing you."

"Ravish" was such a romantic word coming from Oz's lips; now here it was being used again by my new horny suitor. My eyes focused on Tom across the table. He was staring at me like an expectant puppy. I abruptly stood up.

"Let's go."

"What?" he said, as I towered above him.

"You said you want to ravish me." *The Queen of Pussy has spoken!*

"Yes, I—" Tom was stunned.

"Let's go."

Tom threw money on the table. We walked out into the cool night, passing a dark stairwell. I pulled Tom into the shadows. He pushed me back against the brick wall. I heard people walking past the stairwell, oblivious. We kissed eagerly. Our bodies fit well together. I put his hand between my legs, and he gasped with delight when he realized I was fully available to him.

"Let's get a room." I said.

Tom pulled back, looking into my face. He was a good boy at heart.

"Really? I don't want to push you."

It's hard to describe exactly how I felt at that moment. I had endured two years of foreplay with Oz. I wasn't getting laid regularly. I wanted depth but I was willing to lower my standards. I wanted sex *with love* but I was beginning to realize this might be a long wait. Tom was so eager, even euphoric, at the idea of fucking me. And it left me smitten. Granted, it wasn't the startling love connection I had with Oz. But maybe it could grow into something bigger? And even if it didn't, why not get some good action along the way?

We drove to a Days Inn. Tom ponied up his half of the hotel money. The desk clerk told us the only room available didn't have cable.

"Oh we won't be watching TV!" Tom proclaimed energetically.

We all laughed—even the guy in the corner sipping something out of a paper bag laughed.

Tom was quite a technician in the bedroom. He had this way of stimulating my G-spot internally and externally at the same time, which was fantastic. He manipulated me into incredible positions faster than you could mutter "body pretzel." The boy had clearly studied the sexual arts. We made love once and I came easily. He wanted to do it again twenty minutes later. But I was interested in getting to know him, which made me feel a bit self-conscious. We talked but it felt like filler to the main event.

Tom was tremendously sweet and eager. After a second round of lovemaking he told me that Addison was mad at him because he broke off their date that night so he could be with me. *I knew that chick was history once he tasted my world-class pussy!* I shared with him my poly failings in regard to Addison; he laughed.

"Oh, I love that you are telling me this!"

"You do?"

"Sure, poly brings up a lot of feelings, and I am flattered."

"How do you feel when your wife goes out on a date?"

He described the tightening in his chest and his altered heartbeat. I was impressed by his somatic awareness. He was on a rugby team, meditated regularly, and had done therapy. I noted these details, seeing ways we could hopefully bond further.

He asked when he could see me again and could it be for the whole night, a sleepover? This was confusing, since Tom seemed mainly focused on sex. But sleeping side by side, snoring, dreaming, and then waking up together with morning breath, was *so intimate*. I wasn't ready for that, but I told him in a couple of weeks I'd be at a hotel in San Jose for the pagan conference PantheaCon. We could meet there for a sleepover. I'd be ready then.

"I am there, absolutely," he said.

Tom and I had been dating about four weeks when we had our third date. People had told me that in the poly world circumstances could change extremely fast—it was a phenomena, a time dilation in which things could speed up and then suddenly slow back down again, collapsing a six-month relationship into six weeks by sheer speed of its uptake. I was beginning to see what they meant. In just two dates we had bonded and had sex a few times, and we also had a little…not quite a spat…an interchange, maybe?…around how to handle ourselves when Tom was away with his family. He told me that on his family vacation he wouldn't text much. I understood and stopped texting him completely. He wooed me back with a series of passionate texts as he drove up the coast, culminating with "I am going to fuck you like you've never been fucked before in your life." Considering what a slut I had been in earlier years, I was impressed by the proclamation.

The night after he returned, we met for dinner at a sushi restaurant. Tom had borrowed a friend's apartment for the evening. We ordered drinks, and then Tom said, "The apartment isn't available for another hour, so let's just kill time here." I felt stung. Conversing with me was "killing time"?

When we got to the apartment, Tom eagerly guided me to the bedroom. He had planned the menu and executed it with panache. He found places on my body that I didn't even know were erogenous zones. We made love for over an hour, and when he climaxed Tom yelled, "Thank you, OkCupid!"

I rolled over into his arms and said, "Oh, before I leave, let me give you directions to the hotel."

Our February date was in two weeks.

Tom bristled a bit. "Actually that may not work out."

"Oh, really?"

I was confused. He had been thrilled when I'd invited him. Now I could feel his body stiffening.

"I talked with my wife and—you and I would be waking up on Valentine's Day. I have to be with her on Valentine's Day."

I suddenly felt like a poly piece of ass.

"I want to be with Hank and my family on Valentine's Day too. We'd be leaving the hotel that morning."

"Yes, but I absolutely must wake up next to my wife."

I pulled the sheets around me, suddenly not wanting to be nude in front of Tom. He was silent, but I could feel him watching me. It was nice to date a married man. He knew when you were pissed at him. An article I'd read on polyfidelity versus swinging popped into my head. I was now experiencing the contrast of those two different worlds. Tom and his wife went to sex parties together. Their orientation to poly was "just sexual." I was new to poly and still finding my way. But this was a defining moment. *I wanted a lover that would give me a rose on Valentine's Day. I wanted to be loved.* It was clear Tom and his wife were warding that off.

Tom shifted in bed. "Are you angry at me?"

"I am not trying to take your wife's place. Isn't there a way that you can satisfy me and her as well? Valerie has already asked to spend some time with Hank on Valentine's Day."

Tom rolled away from me.

"No, I can't do that."

"Why?"

"Because Valentine's Day is special it's—"

"—for people you love?" I added.

"Yes. It's for people you love."

There was an awkward pause. I started dressing. Tom sat up in bed watching me.

"Grace, the last thing I was thinking about when I got into poly was falling in love."

His tone annoyed me. He was like a banker—all friendly when you are depositing money but suddenly remote when you want a loan.

"Okay, I understand."

I put on my dress.

"You are a really nice woman."

Oh, go to hell.

I was dressed. I turned to face him.

"I feel like a piece of ass."

"I am sorry, Grace. We want different things."

"Yes, we do."

I put on my jean jacket and picked up my purse.

"Let's talk tomorrow."

"No, I don't think so," I said.

"Are you dumping me?"

"Yes. I think I am done. It was nice meeting you."

Then I left. I got in my car and started to drive—and cry. This had opened the dark pit of my insecurities. At first it had been so exciting to think of getting laid. But now I remembered how empty the dating world could be. Oz had inspired me to open my marriage because of the depth of love he had for me; I had felt memorized and adored by him. Vacuous sex marathons with random men were not going to fulfill me. I needed to feel special with a man, not just like the latest flavor of ass.

When I got home Hank was reading on the couch. I came in and sat across from him. He looked up from his book.

"Are you okay?"

"I am in so much pain trying to get what I need." My voice choked with sobs, I could barely get the words out. "You stopped having sex with me. Now I'm at the mercy of all these creeps."

It had been so long since I'd been this raw. But poly was a different realm of experience, a grand experiment that asked us to shed all artifice.

Hank removed his reading glasses, his eyes filled with concern. I could see that he wanted to take away my pain and was now realizing that he had become a source of it. Over the years there were many times Hank had withdrawn from me. I would laugh it off. But I couldn't make light of it tonight. Hank was the person who most fully understood me. He understood how devastated I had been when my father rejected me again. It occurred to me that I had never let him know how much pain I felt over our sex life.

"I am so sorry," Hank said, and then he started to sob in a way I had not seen him cry in decades. Seeing my pain overwhelmed him; our mission had been to heal each other and somehow we had stopped short. I felt sad for the both of us.

"It's okay," I said, clutching his hand.

His body was quaking with sobs. I was crying too. We sat next to each not saying much, holding hands. I loved him so much. What could a person do? Relationships had their seasons—it wasn't anyone's fault.

I felt so much tenderness toward Hank that night, seeing him so raw. I wanted to talk to him more about it, so about a month later I mentioned this cathartic moment to Hank. He couldn't remember it.

"When did I cry?" he asked.

I took it in with great sadness. I was beginning to fully comprehend how Hank could "put away" overwhelming emotions in his psyche. Somewhere along the way, he had locked away our sex life. The grief I felt over this was large.

Post-Tom, I was pretty gloomy. I landed on my feet—but just barely. My friends surrounded me like an emotional SWAT team. A week after my nightmare date, Freya came over to lounge outside, drink red wine, and eat large amounts of chocolate.

As we were talking, Valerie and Hank returned from a hike with Tallulah and Merlin. We had introduced Valerie to the kids a couple weeks ago. The kids had seemed to attach to Valerie in a similar way as they'd accepted Freya into their lives: another Auntie to spend time with. We told the kids that Valerie was Hank's "special friend." We did not want to tell them they were dating.

I was happy about the seamless way Valerie had become a part of our family life in five short months. She was my first "gift" in the world of poly, becoming a friend and coach in my preparations for entering the dating scene. One afternoon we had lunch together and discussed everything from Hank's quirks, our lacking relationships with our fathers, and the current dating etiquette for handling issues of safe sex. Valerie coached me like a close friend or sister. In fact, that was what this new connection felt like to me: a sister-in-law. We were brought together by a mutual person that we both loved and were determined to share—without stepping on each other's toes over him. Poly seemed like another opportunity to have a chosen family that could benefit kids.

The kids squealed with delight when they saw Freya, hugging her and then eating our chocolate. Sweet tooths satisfied, Tallulah and Merlin grabbed Valerie, pulling her upstairs to show her an art project they'd completed. Then Hank asked me if he could drive Valerie to a dance class she was taking. The kids came down and announced that they wanted to go with Valerie and Daddy. So they all left. Freya and I sipped our Shiraz.

"Hank and Valerie are celebrating their five-month anniversary," I said a bit dourly.

"That's nice," Freya said.

"Yeah, I am so happy for them," I said weakly.

"I can see that," Freya added, then we both started laughing.

"I've become a cautionary tale," I moaned. "I can hear people talking '...*SHE* opened the marriage and then *HE* fell in love and *SHE—well...it's sad*,'" I shook my head. Freya chuckled.

It was Saturday afternoon and technically it was my date night. But I had no one to use it with. Aurora had organized a poly meet-up: a dive-bar tour of the Mission District. She texted, asking if I was coming. Freya encouraged me to go. She had a hot date herself and would be abandoning me shortly. I was on the fence. I was feeling cynical, but the live aspect of the night was appealing. No long-winded e-mails posing for each other, just real-time conversing and immediate confirmation of whether he had a nice ass. I decided to go for it.

I showed up at the dive bar wearing a super-cleavage pink dress and sporting a leopard-print umbrella, to protect me from the rain. The bar at Sixteenth Street and Valencia was half full. I walked through it twice but couldn't find Aurora. I went outside and called her on my cell phone, standing in the drizzle. I contemplated heading back home to curl up with my kids and watch a movie. That was the great thing about dating with kids and a husband: the action had to be good because you had better at home.

I turned to go when Aurora came up and wrapped her arms around me. She led me into the bar. There were two younger men in their twenties, looking like bewildered deer on the edge of a slope. Then there was a dude my age. He had thick-rimmed Clark Kent–type glasses and a lovely British accent. Soon I was drinking whiskey and chatting up the boys. I loved the imbalanced gender ratio. I wasn't sure who would be the lucky winner of—drum roll, please—a make-out session with me.

We switched to the next bar on the tour. Clark Kent asked if he could share my leopard umbrella. By the third bar, Clark was sidling up to me trying to edge out his competitors. I felt like I had to breast-feed the younger boys through sophisticated conversation. I liked Clark Kent; he had life experience. But then he started bragging about some twenty-four-year-old chick he was bagging regularly. It was embarrassing to see the middle-aged reflection of myself, although I had come down from my younger-man fetish. By the fourth bar he texted me, "If I buy you a drink will you promise to talk only to me?" Nice, erudite flirting. I texted back that for the price of a martini he would buy "total exclusivity."

We ended up ditching everyone, giggling under my umbrella and skipping through the rain till we got to my car.

"May I join you for a bit inside your vehicle?"

The British accent was moistening my loins. We slipped inside and sat next to each other on the front seat. Clark made me laugh telling stories about his wife's verbally autistic, unemployed boy-friend. He was mystified as to why his wife was "completely enam-ored by him." Talk subsided, then Clark leaned in for a deep kiss. Raindrops sounded like chimes as they fell on the car roof. We started to touch each other more frantically, zippers unzipping, buttons flicked open. After twenty minutes I told Clark to take me to his apartment—*now*.

Clark stuttered, "I have an agreement with my wife that we can't use the apartment for women I meet—and I have to clear sex with her."

I told Clark I'd split a hotel room. He quickly dialed his wife—*who didn't answer!* Clark looked at me apologetically.

"Can I take you out tomorrow? I really like you."

Good Goddess, this dude clearly doesn't have offspring.

I tried to explain, "I am free for another three hours—that's the window!"

I wanted sex *now.* Clark called his wife again—then texted her—but to no avail.

After Tom, I had a metallic ring of protection around my heart. I liked Clark, but his talk about bedding twentysomething babes made me apprehensive. The only time I ever wanted *just sex* was after a few drinks, with a charming attractive man that I'd likely never see again—a one-off. I accepted defeat and decided to go home to my vibrator.

When I arrived home, everyone was asleep, snuggled in our king bed. I decided to hunker down in Tallulah's room, but I was so wired that I couldn't sleep. I got my tarot deck and fanned the cards out facedown. I pulled three cards on my currently sucky love life.

"What will happen in the next month?" I asked.

I got the Justice card first; this implied that things were happening as they should, and that justice would prevail. Then I got the Lovers card; good…but I was having lovers but no success. Then I got Two of Wands reversed—which usually means more suckage. Yet, I was confused given the position of the card. I flipped open my reference book. What I read there sent a chill down my spine.

Expect the unexpected—a long-desired love is now available, the fairy tale ending manifests.

I gasped. *Could this be about Oz?* I imagined him way up the hillside in his house—breathing. *Was he still alive? Did he really exist or had I dreamed him?* I had not seen him for months. *What did I not expect?*

Chapter 9

Dark Tuesday began like any other lousy day. At first I thought it was going to be your garden-variety general bad day, when about halfway through it morphed into a *seriously bad day*. I felt like one of those hospital workers who assume they are dealing with a typical infection, then realize they have on their hands bacteria ready to eat the skin off a corpse—way past their worst expectations.

I had been dating in the poly world about five months—and let's just say things weren't quite going my way, but I was hanging in. After the Tom debacle, I had a long talk with Aurora. I told her with a sneer about Tom's shallow sexual pursuits. She encouraged me not to judge, that as long as Tom was honest with the women he was treating like pieces of ass on a conveyor belt, it was all within the good poly dating practices.

As much as I respected Aurora, I couldn't agree. I had evolved a slightly different mindset. I had always felt that it was one thing to be sex positive and another thing to be treated rudely—whether in a poly relationship or not. I realized that, in poly, a gal could be easily tricked into the illusion that boorish behavior was all just "good jolly poly." Having a *sanctioned* steady flow of ass—multiple partners not only allowable but the jealousy typically associated with it *unallowable*—could be the perfect storm for an unsophisticated man to make sexist, rude blunders.

If Tom had told me point-blank on date one that he had little interest in my brain and heart, and just wanted some good pussy, I would have declined. Though he was likely well-intentioned, Tom was over his head in a situation that called for delicacy and finesse.

But Aurora did have some good advice. She told me to avoid profiles that talked about swinging and sex parties and to look for the phrase "polyfidelity." People practicing polyfidelity were looking for deeper long-term commitments within their multiple-relationship lifestyles.

After our talk, I scanned OkCupid for an hour. I was determined to find an available poly dude who wasn't a freak. I decided to reread the profile of Bobby Z, who had popped up as a match months ago. He lived about fifteen minutes away and was into polyfidelity. I e-mailed him, and an hour later he responded. He was out of his mind happy that I'd contacted him. He said he'd noticed me months ago when I first posted my profile but that the Universe warned him that I wasn't ready to meet him. He had decided to wait till I reached out to him. I liked his psychic vibe. We booked a date. I was like an old cattle rancher: if his teeth looked clean I'd purchase.

We met at Cyclops Cave, which had become "my bar." I got there a few minutes early. Right on the dot Bobby Z walked in. He carried a bouquet of organic vegetables: purple cauliflower, radishes, and several bunches of kale. *Points for a creative touch!* He had noted in my profile that I loved vegetables. I commented on the bouquet.

He replied, "You said you wanted to be wooed, so I am wooing you."

We got some drinks and sat down. He listened well and asked all the right questions. He was psychologically adept. We discussed our families of origin and empathized with each other. Bobby Z had had a long career as a mime; when he got up to order more drinks I noted how he moved with a fluid awareness. He had two other girlfriends. But the way he talked about them was really nice. He didn't seem weird about it. (Although I had to admit my weird meter had recalibrated—it took quite a zinger to set off the alarm. I was beginning to wonder if I'd altered my standards and had transformed to the point of having really low expectations—and it had happened so slowly I hadn't noticed. Was poly just a really bad dating scenario? Four months ago I was searching for a stellar man the caliber of Oz; now I'd settle for a guy who'd buy me a drink and not comment on my tits till date two.) But even with these questions swimming in my head I was charmed by Bobby Z. After an hour of talking and a few kisses, I was sold.

After our initial meeting at Cyclops Cave, we had two dates within ten days. Bobby Z continued to be charming…but something started to feel off. On date three he told me he was falling in love with me—which was nice. After all, I am a girl whose type is stalker. But it also felt like Bobby Z was too enthused to know me well enough to declare his affections. Now I know that sounds odd and even debatable—a best friend, upon hearing such a declaration, would say with real positivity, "But you know you're a catch!" And it's true: I am a nice gal. But it was as if someone knowing me for thirty minutes had suddenly wanted to buy a condominium together in Tahoe. *Why?* I was a virtual stranger.

Even for me—a self-proclaimed glutton for attention riddled with low self-esteem and longing for sexual encounters—it was too much too soon. I wanted to tell him, *Dude—make me work for it! At least interrogate me for ten minutes before you decide you're in love with me!* The whole thing felt like "love lite"—a low-calorie diet love, a love that left you hungry and creeping down the back stairs at three a.m. to raid the refrigerator. I mean, with poly how hard is it to get on someone's top-five list—was this really an achievement? In poly you weren't *the one*, you were *one of the five*. One of the five greatest chicks your new man loved to bang. The whole thought of it made my body sag with despair. It just didn't hold much allure.

At high noon on Dark Tuesday I realized with remorse that I was not achieving my goal to supplement my life with a fantastic man. I felt the magnetic pull toward Oz, yet again. I thought of our promised six-month check-in. That was back in October; it was now February. I had *promised* myself I'd be over him within six months. I knew I would be over him, like you know you are going to lose those pesky five pounds you acquired over Thanksgiving and Christmas—those handful of pounds that linger like a friendly layer of cottage cheese where your hamstrings meet your ass; what Pilates instructors call "the gluteal fold." Now you look in the mirror and those unwelcome pounds, dauntingly stubborn, wave back at you, another reminder of how your whole existence is barely within your control.

I fantasized about running into Oz at the school auction in March. I imagined myself fluttering like a vivacious social butterfly. "Oh! What a nice surprise to see you," I'd say, chatting him up casually, while internally I'd be completely unmoved because I'd be with a new, available man—I'd be fulfilled. *I was supremely confident that I would triumph.*

Five months ago I had entered the dating scene with ebullient optimism and excitement to get laid. But the glimmer had worn off. I felt like a piece of (cottage cheese) ass in the dating trenches. When I had started out, it was enough to get attention and sex. But I was beginning to realize I wanted so much more. I wanted that glorious feeling of being in love, to be fascinated to hear every little thing about each other and take care of each other. In short, I wanted everything I had with Oz but in an available man. But all I was finding was an abundance of horny guys and shallow connections.

It was becoming clear to me that I wasn't just sex-starved. Poly was most thrilling when it held the possibility of having Oz. The prize of a bunch of horny men wanting me was losing its appeal fast. I was hard up trying to find the right lover. Actually, "hard up" was being generous—*humiliated* was putting a positive spin on it. I was feeling all Glenn Close in *Fatal Attraction*, curled up in my bed, dirty plates by my side, *Oprah* blaring in the background.

My cell phone was lying by my side. It felt like a conduit to love. I picked up the magical listening device. The smooth metallic case felt almost soft and slippery in my hand. *What would I say if I were actually going to text Oz—two months early?* I cringed. I put down the phone and stared at the ceiling. I knew this whole thing with Oz wasn't going to work out. All my friends and even Hank had tried to get me off the smack. Just last week Hank had said to me gently, "He has more in common with his wife than he does with you. They're corporate types, they think alike. They aren't going to open their marriage."

I had heard through the grapevine that Oz was working with Lily, our poly counselor. I hoped that Susan might be willing to open their marriage—but if this weren't so, I had to move on. Poly could not be one sided. Susan had to give her full consent, otherwise it was cheating. But it was so unlikely that this would happen. I had to find a poly lover who was similar to Oz. This was turning out to be a tall order, but I wanted to get on with getting on. What I needed right now was a final rejection from Oz, a confirmation from the source—I needed to hear Oz say that he had officially and permanently closed the door on the idea of us being lovers. Then I could move on.

I picked up my cell phone and typed out his name. A blank bubble appeared on my little screen. I paused again. I had dreamed of texting Oz so often in the last four months that this was the farthest I'd gotten. I could feel my heart beating rapidly.

I sat up and started quickly pressing the letters with my forefinger. *I'll keep it neutral and chirpy,* I thought to myself. I typed.

I am at a crossroads and wanted to check in.

How would that play? I wondered. I felt racy and daring. I looked at the tiny viewer window that held my sentence, like a miniature canoe holding little words that seemed monstrously large. I let my finger linger above the send button, gently rubbing it, playing chicken, and knowing I couldn't really do it. Then I felt a slight almost spasmodic impulsive pressure as my fingertip depressed and—*Oh My Goddess—it was sent.* I sent it! I felt like the Lexington minuteman whose musket accidentally discharged, firing the shot that would be heard around the world. *What had I just done?* Now the revolution had begun. I lay back on the pillows on my bed and stared at the ceiling. *What would happen next?* I wanted Oz to text back, "Susan and I are so grateful to hear from you. Can we meet for dinner and plan our new poly life together?" Clearly I was deranged. *A rejection was on its way.*

After a few moments I forced myself to sit up. I swung my legs around and placed my feet on the floor. I looked around the room at the dishes, dirty laundry on the floor, the dreaded cell phone. I needed new scenery. I decided to go downstairs and maul my husband. This was perhaps the greatest gift of marital life: *you have someone to blame.*

I felt a little bit like pictures I'd seen of Elizabeth Taylor when she was boozing it up with Richard Burton—once glamorous and now somehow off, about to reel out of control. When I was a kid I read in *Life* magazine about a reporter who had interviewed Burton when he and Elizabeth Taylor had first met on the set of *Cleopatra* and were carrying on like two rabbits in heat. Elizabeth had come to the balcony overlooking the terrace where Burton and the reporter were sitting. She *whined* for him to get his sorry alcoholic ass upstairs and fuck her. You've just *got* to admire this in a woman.

Almost from the moment we exit the vaginal canal we're told in a thousand different ways to be *a Lady, a nice girl, a sweet little thing.* Don't burp. Wash your armpits, sit up straight, smile, repress your anger, and lose at tennis. Good Goddess, at that moment Elizabeth Taylor should have been given a lifetime achievement award for being sloppy drunk and pussy focused.

As I came downstairs, swaying from a slight sugar high, I spotted Hank in the living room texting Valerie. I was wearing my not-even-trying-to-be-pretty sweats that made my ass look bulbous. I had a stain on my shirt from a recent sugar indulgence. My whole demeanor and attire said, *Go ahead* and *tell me to put on a cute outfit. I'll chew through the largest artery in your neck.* Our loft-like living room felt offensively expansive. I looked around at the clean open space as I waddled like a dumpy Cleopatra to the center of the room.

Sunlight poured into the bay of floor-to-ceiling windows at the apex of the room, where Hank had designed a little stage that was flanked by twenty-foot-tall sheets of glass that looked out to the garden. The sun was jarring in contrast to my mood. It made me feel like a vampire rolling out of her coffin. Hank put his cell phone by his side. I glared at him as I plopped down in our Hans Wegner papa bear chair that frequently reminded me of Captain Kirk's seat on the starship *Enterprise*, with its majestic arms and slight recline. I looked over at Hank and smiled a little sarcastic smirk. Hank returned my gaze, the deer checking out the lion, seeming to wonder, *Can I get away?*

I've got to hand it to Hank; he really pulls these situations off nicely. He had the gift of the married man who'd been handling a woman through pregnancies, estrogen outbreaks, and generalized female angst for a good decade or two. I could see him in another twenty years at a bar, sipping a beer with his future son-in-law, "Son, when your woman is hormonal or just gets that wild-eyed look, remain calm—you can and will ride it out." He had seen me in this state before.

But this time was worse than the other times. I was on a bender—reckless with despair. I felt like I'd surpassed Elizabeth Taylor in her petulant plea to Burton; I'd even surpassed her in sexual frustration in her portrayal of Maggie in *Cat on a Hot Tin Roof*. I'd played Tennessee Williams's Maggie the Cat in my acting days, performed her famous nonstop trill of an opening monologue, which was more like an aria than a speech. I'd played the role so well, the highly sexed girl rebuffed by her husband, oozing with heat and desire.

But that day was done. I was now Liz twenty years later, too much bitterness with Burton, that pickled pompous bastard who caused her to overeat and become a chubby shell of her violet-eyed self. I was Liz in *Who's Afraid of Virginia Woolf?*—furious and mean didn't even begin to encompass where I'd landed. I was practically burping and slurring as I gazed at Hank, a sneer playing across my lips.

"How's Valerie?" This was not a question; it was a sarcastic harpoon flying through the air ready to sink into Hank's chest.

"She's good." Hank was calm.

Oh, so it's like that? Fine, pretend to ignore the bubbling rage seething beneath my ugly surface.

"It must be nice having regular sex."

I was so unsheathed and nude in my self-pity. Welcome to one of the many Top Ten Most Miserable Moments of my life. If my life were a movie, this would be the scene where you'd pause the video to augment the moment with carbohydrates. You'd say to your husband, "I knew the whole thing would blow up in her face," as you spooned some Ben & Jerry's Chubby Hubby into your mouth, contented that this wasn't your drama, your nightmare. I imagined myself telling my friends about the current scene unfolding. They would listen and coo with empathy, hiding their smugness. They'd think, "Wow, Grace's life is a real train wreck." I was that person people discuss at cocktail parties, the person who dared to veer off the beaten path and had failed miserably, the renegade who gets heartily trounced for daring to do it differently. People love these stories; it makes them feel superior in their predictably complacent lives.

I eyed Hank. "I am so angry at you. You withdraw from me. I am so fed up that we don't have sex."

While I was fuming, I recalled the night a few weeks ago when I had hired a babysitter so Hank and I could have some time alone. We tried to be amorous, but I had felt like I was talking someone into a doubtful real estate investment. Hank confessed to me, "I feel like I'm cheating on Valerie." *Can you believe the irony of that?* In the beginning we saw ourselves continuing to have sex with each other, but then I realized I had been completely usurped. Why couldn't Hank and I have great, passionate sex? I loved him so much. Our relationship had the depth, so why couldn't we have the passion too?

"I hate that we don't have sex," I repeated redundantly.

I started a monologue. It was startling, even spectacular, in its head-first leap down the black hole of misery. The dire situation reminded me of a story about someone's husband who would *beg* his wife for a hand job. They had two kids under the age of four, and that was the most he could expect to get. It was like, "Baby, will you please touch my dick so I know it's still there and doesn't just exist in my imagination?" *I could more than relate.*

Why had I chosen a man who withheld sex from me? Me, Ms. Hornypants, had chosen a man who needed vast amounts of alone time and habitually withdrew. *How did I get here? I don't deserve this!* I was the woman in my mother's group who'd dragged my husband to a "Tantra Art of Lovemaking" weekend workshop when Tallulah was six months old. All the other husbands in that group thought I was a hero. At our barbecues they would nod at me with respectful awe. I could read their minds: "That girl is trying to get it on with her man. Between leaky breasts and baby spit-up, she still has game." They practically took their hats off and genuflected when I entered the room.

But my own man was burdened by my sex drive and, to add insult to injury, was happily getting it on with another woman, leaving me out in the cold with a bunch of shallow, horny poly bastards. *Oh the angst, the ongoing humiliation!* It made me want a new life, with a fresh set of problems.

I continued my monologue. Hank's calm gaze soothed me. Occasionally his cell phone would ding with a sexy little text from Valerie. But the boy didn't move a muscle. His gaze was continuous and unbroken as if his life depended on it—*which it did.* Although I was calming down, one wrong move, one utterance of "Oh, it's Valerie, can I just get this?" and that boy's neck would have been half eaten. He listened, completely focused on me.

"I just don't know about Bobby Z. I want to like him but I just don't feel the enthusiasm."

"There's no reason for you to date someone you don't feel enthusiastic about."

I nodded.

"I am just not meeting men I like. I want a man like Oz. I want someone who is really interested in who I am."

Hank's eyes were gentle pools of empathy. He told me to be patient.

"You want filet mignon and you are surrounded by hamburgers. Hamburgers are easy— pull into any fast-food joint and you can get a hamburger. But you want a gourmet meal. You've got to be willing to wait."

I nodded again. I felt like a tiny forlorn babe needing guidance.

"What should I do about Bobby Z?"

It felt odd but also correct to be receiving counsel from Hank about my love life.

He spoke with assurance, "Cancel. You are a beautiful woman. You'll find what you're looking for."

I could tell by his demeanor that Hank felt guilty. Somewhere inside he knew he had not put enough effort into making our sex life work. He had let me be the one to do all the personal growth; now he was dealing with my anger. It was unclear to me why we stopped having sex. *How can you live with someone for twenty-five years and not fully understand him?* Sometimes Hank's psyche felt like a labyrinth to me—there were so many hidden passages and unexpected trap doors.

Hank continued, "If you aren't feeling interested, then trust yourself. There's no reason for you to compromise."

More nodding, a mute zombie who needed step-by-step directions. I decided to call Bobby Z and break it off before our next date in two days. We were planning on biking around Inspiration Point. My fluff and stuff had been kicked out of me. If we were biking Misery Lane—maybe—but I just couldn't muster the enthusiasm.

As I climbed the stairs to my bedroom I heard Hank clicking a text on his cell phone, probably to Valerie. *Goddess, would I find someone I felt equally as enthused about?* When I started out on my poly odyssey this was a given, but now I was realizing my love with Oz was one of those lifetime rarities. It might be a long wait to make a connection like that again.

Forty-five minutes later I drove over the bridge into San Francisco. Somehow I had collected myself, cleaned up, and got my happy-trainer face on. Once a week I went into the city to train a group of women living in a halfway house. They were all victims of domestic violence from their families or husbands. I had looked for a job like this, working with trauma survivors. I felt passionate about helping women who had survived abuse, having been down that road myself with my stepfather. And having done so much work to heal myself, I had an innate ability to uplift and inspire the under-dogs of the world. I had designed them a state-of-the-art gym and showed up at the house weekly with unbounded enthusiasm. But today, feeling so wacked myself, I could barely mobilize the energy to be the health and wellness gal.

As I drove, I looked at the San Francisco skyline. The buildings boldly contrasted the clear blue sky. It made me feel weepy. It reminded me of the Emerald City, so filled with promise and expectation. At that moment, gazing at the Emerald City, I heard my cell phone ding. I was driving Hank's pickup truck with its rugged, beat-up seats. My cell phone lay on the car seat next to me like a basket filled with snakes. I looked at it with dread; I could see Oz's name on the screen.

Five minutes later I parked in front of the group home, picked up my phone, and read the text. Oz wrote that he was "focusing on his marriage" and he couldn't have any contact with me. I was oddly relieved. *There's your answer. It's over. Get on with your life.*

I felt that elated numb feeling when you get bad news you half expected. I'd become like a righteously grim pilgrim rolling up my starched sleeves to continue the inexorable march to the grave. Somehow I made it through my shift. I drove home and ate dinner with my kids, gave them a bath, poured an extra glass of Chardonnay, and was in bed by nine p.m., relieved that at least life had a restart button you could press at the end of those miserable dark days you want so thankfully to come to an end.

At two a.m. I woke with a start. I felt an oppressive heaviness in my chest. *Good Goddess, I used to be able to bury my feelings if I overate and drank a half bottle of Chardonnay.* I lay in bed, hearing Hank's gentle snore with each intake of breath. I knew what I needed to do: go downstairs and open the journal on my computer titled "Do Not Read. ~Do Not Print." Of course, this will be the first journal that my ancestors will open and print years after my death. It will confirm what they already knew—*yes, mental illness runs in the family.* With repulsed horror they'll wade through the pitiful, verbose entries. I'll be thankful I'm dead.

I sat at my computer and sobbed and wrote, wrote and sobbed. I let myself do this from time to time and find it quite helpful to swim, gulp, then choke on my waves of self-pity. As if lancing a wound, I let loose my rage at Hank, all the pus and anger flowing unedited:

> I hate Hank for withdrawing from me! I hate Oz—because—because I just fucking do. I hate everyone—except my kids, Freya, and maybe one or two of my clients. But I hate everyone else.

It was a state of mind best hidden from the world. This is the part of me that enjoys when those A-game people who sail through life trip and fall and skin their chins—and get a nasty infection, and then their antibiotics give them a yeast infection. Every pore in my body was oozing schadenfreude.

After an hour, I felt somewhat cleansed—still depressed but slightly more functional. I collected the handful of mucus-filled tissues. I felt relief. On a whim I decided to check my e-mail. My tired eyes perused my messages, which were overwhelmingly junk mail. Then my eye tripped over a message and returned startled. It was his name, the mere utterance of which sent a warm thrill through my veins: *Oz had e-mailed me!* It sat in my inbox a glistening jewel in a sea of spam. Incredulously I opened it and read:

> Got an affidavit for limited engagement. I would love to talk with you on the phone. Please email or text your availability. I love you with all of my heart. Oz

I gasped. A white dove burst from the dark cave of my chest. Then I sat frozen, my muscles in near rigor mortis for at least five minutes staring at his words. My fingers were cupped over my mouth, like a *Jane Eyre* character postcoital, stunned, my body shivering with bewilderment and wonder. A possible new world had opened. *What to do?* I suddenly felt so fragile. I didn't want to get into another crazy roller coaster ride pining for Oz. I also needed to talk to Susan. I had to speak directly to her and find out if she was really open to Oz and me having any contact.

Finally my fingers tapped out an e-mail telling Oz how much I loved him and making one thing clear:

> If this is going to work I need to talk with Susan. Is she available to have tea? That's the next step for me.

I signed off, then pressed send and went back to bed. It took me a while to fall back to sleep. I tossed and turned in bed for several hours—every fiber of my being awake with the possibilities.

Chapter 10

I was scared. Was the crazy ride starting again? When Oz and I parted ways back in October I told him I wanted off of the cortisol roller coaster. My marriage was open and I had clearance to talk to Oz, but as far as I knew, he was still forbidden to have any contact with me. One of the main reasons I wanted to do poly was to avoid lying and hiding. I felt that it was unhealthy to hide. It wasn't poly if one partner was in the dark.

Whenever I saw Oz at the school while dropping my kids off, I would be filled with adrenalin, my heart would pound, and my hands would shake. I had read a study on the effects of cortisol, the fight-or-flight hormone, and the contrasting hormone, oxytocin. Cortisol is great when you're being chased by a saber-toothed tiger, but if too much cortisol is present it destroys cells and weakens our immune systems.

I wanted oxytocin, *the love hormone*. It is what flows through a mother's body as she holds her baby to breastfeed and what's present when we orgasm. In October, I wrote Oz saying that I needed ninety percent oxytocin in my relationships.

Ten percent of cortisol is good to feel stimulated, but hiding this friendship creates too many giddy highs followed by excruciating lows. I need everything to be out in the open.

That was four months ago, and now that we were scheduling a phone call I felt apprehensive. I did not want to backslide. Was this friendship just a bad flashback to my attempts to win a father? Was this a love that required me to constantly perform to win it? In the last few months, while dating again, I had realized that the love Oz and I shared was rare and would be hard to replace. But I didn't want drama—all parties had to be in agreement to move forward.

I had met poly people who had inspired me. What I had found most striking in the world of poly was the creativity in constructing relationships, and the lack of shame in seeking fulfillment of needs. In my poly support group, each person had a different setup that responded to his or her unique needs for attention, sex, or being adored. There was an "anything goes" philosophy, so long as everyone was in agreement. For instance, there were Darlene and Richard and Naomi, who lived in a one-bedroom flat and together ran an upholstery business. Then Steve and Jon, who were madly in love and had been dating for six years but who also happened to be legally married to women who didn't mind.

I was open to different scenarios as long as it felt good to all parties. If Oz and I were allowed to be platonic friends, perhaps then I could supplement that friendship with sexual encounters. I was trying to patch together a situation that worked for me and honored other people's boundaries. But the one thing I was absolutely sure of was that hiding and lying was not what I was looking for.

It was clear to me that my next step was talking to Susan. I didn't want Oz to be our go-between anymore; it was a bad game of telephone. I wasn't getting the straight dope. I wanted to hear directly from her. It was with this intention that I e-mailed her a request to meet with me.

I was pretty sure I had reached my intake capacity for nerve-racking ordeals as I hit SEND and stared pathetically at my inbox. And then I remembered: I had a date. I reread the e-mail from two days ago, hoping it would steer my emotions in a different direction.

Hey, Sweetie!
I just finished watching one of your shows online. It was fantastic. I want to learn more about your writing on our bike ride. I bought you a water bottle and an extra tire tube. Do you need anything else?

I never canceled the bike-ride date with Bobby Z, even though Hank had encouraged me to do so after our talk on Dark Tuesday. What kind of ungrateful bitch cancels after such a nice e-mail? Hadn't I asked the Universe to deliver me a guy who was genuine and kind—not just hustling me into bed? I had heard my own motherly advice in my head, *You asked for a love connection that was primarily oxytocin, so go on another date with him.*

When I opened my front door, there was Bobby Z looking svelte in his biking shorts.

"Hi, gorgeous!" he said.

We hugged. And for a long second I had the urge to call off the bike ride and drag him by his spandex waistband to the couch so we could make out. He seemed cuddly, like a guy you could languidly kiss for hours. But my internal mother prodded me out the door.

We drove to Inspiration Point in his Volkswagen bus with a DIY wooden bicycle rack on top. As he filled my bike tires with air, he accidentally caused a flat when he pulled out the pump latch too abruptly. But he calmly went to the edge of the road, and within moments he flagged down a cyclist who, with great kindness, gave us a tire tube. I admired Bobby's style. He was one of those people who seemed to be in harmony with his surroundings.

Being with Bobby Z was like being in a Monet painting in his blue phase. Everything was watery and flowing. I felt the oxytocin streaming through my veins. I appreciated Bobby Z's attentiveness. He asked me to ride ahead of him, not to check out my ass (although he probably did that too) but to assess the height of my bike seat. He said my hips were shifting too much, and we stopped so he could adjust my bike. It was lovely to feel so cared for.

As Bobby Z adjusted my bike, I noticed that Oz had texted me. Susan had gotten my e-mail and would reply soon. Oz's text gave me a slight adrenalin surge as I floated in the water lilies. *Do I really need this crazy Oz thing?* I wondered. The contrast in my body was worth noting. If Bobby Z was a Monet painting, my world with Oz was like a Picasso, filled with odd transfixing portraits in which women's heads were off kilter and their lips an inch away from their jaws. The what-will-happen-next nature of our relationship was edgy, even captivating, but my connection to Oz sometimes felt psychologically askew and even creepy. Who needed that? I really needed some solidarity, not a grueling dating game of Russian roulette. I turned off my iPhone and shoved it into my pocket. I watched Bobby Z's sinewy muscles as he adjusted my saddle, my mind conjuring images of us entwined in bed.

After our ride, Bobby Z and I went to Cyclops Cave to drink and make out. The bartender was wearing a wifebeater tank and sporting tattoos on his massive arm muscles. As he placed our cocktails on the bar, Bobby Z tipped an imaginary top hat to him. The bartender smirked as Bobby Z and I carried our drinks to the table. Then Bobby Z's phone rang. It was one of his girlfriends. He took his call in the hallway by the bathrooms, then returned a moment later. As he walked to the table he mimed seeing a flower, plucking it, and offering it to me. Evidently this was part of his shtick—he clearly loved the art of miming—and yet he reminded me a bit of a high-school boy one misstep from cool, a boy unable to resist telling the dorky joke that would unwittingly repel the pussy he so desired. Internally I shook my head, then called upon my Viola Spolin training and plucked an imaginary flower from thin air; I held it with panache between my teeth like a flamenco dancer.

Bobby grinned as he sat down. We started talking about Daoism, which is close in philosophy to Witchcraft. As we shared our similar spiritual philosophies, I realized that he was everything I had asked for.

When he brought me home, I didn't even mind that he was heading off on a date with one of his other girlfriends. He looked genuinely sad, as if leaving me was hugely difficult. My ego was assuaged... And yet, as I watched his van pull away, all I could think about was Oz. *Good Lilith, will I ever get over the big O?*

The looming conversation with Susan seemed messy verging on ugly. My poly friend Alex had slightly disapproved of the situation when I told him about Oz and his wife. He gently warned me of people who claim to be poly but are actually just snooping for an easy lay. Alex counseled me to look for people who were genuinely poly. Bobby Z seemed to embody the poly philosophy that first excited me. Even though he had other lovers, I felt he could go deep with me in an authentic and caring way. I also liked his innately feminist take on my life. When I told him about my dearth of getting laid with Hank, he related to it—not from a place of machismo but a genuine sense of compassion.

But Alex had worried unnecessarily about Susan's intentions. That night I received a reply from Susan. It was my impression that she had no interest in doing polyamory—and that she was in immense pain. I felt shocked and saddened. I was thankful I had reached out to her. In the past year when I talked with Oz, he would tell me how great things were in his marriage and that it had "never been better." Perhaps this was true from his perspective. I had envisioned that they were going through a similar process to what Hank and I were having: stressful, yet illuminating and causing positive change. I imagined it would feel awful having my spouse ask me to open our relationship if it frightened me or went against my value system. I did not want to be a part of coercing someone. I e-mailed Oz telling him I had to say good-bye.

Oz called me immediately. He was at work and took his phone outside.

"Please, don't go."

"But Susan doesn't want this, and she's in so much pain."

"I love her very much, but I can't stop loving you. I've tried to do what society wants me to do, and what Susan wants me to, do but I just can't stop loving you."

I didn't know what to say.

Oz went on, "Will you stay for a while? I have clearance to talk to you on the phone. Please stay—I want to try and see if Susan will allow us to be friends."

I felt myself hesitating, trying to find the energy to say good-bye, yet wondering if perhaps this was a better next step. It felt devastating to hear of Susan's pain, but trying to give Oz up and be back in the same place six months later also felt wrong.

"Alright," I answered. "I won't go away."

But internally I was sure this would not work. Perhaps I could use the time to shore up enough energy to leave once and for all.

I thought about all this as I drove to PantheaCon, the conference I had invited Tom to. It had been little more than two weeks since I dumped Tom, made out with Clark Kent, and had three dates with Bobby Z. Time was accelerating again, and I was in a whole new era—some conclusion was about to happen with Oz. And I knew it was likely to be a loss. But I felt high in this state of letting go; I felt righteous, like a spiritual zealot. I would give up Oz and make amends to Susan. I would offer her free Pilates sessions—an idea I soon abandoned because I recognized she probably would not want to be in the same room with me. I was stoned on contact with Oz. But I knew the ax would fall soon, like a solider must feel as a surgeon prepares to saw off his gangrenous arm. I would do it. It would hurt, but giving up Oz was the right thing to do.

I walked into the hotel lobby filled with pagans in full Earth-worshipping regalia. That evening I went to a women's full-moon ritual, then holed up with some pals in our hotel room to drink red wine and gab. The next morning I strolled through the pagan mall filled with vendors selling tools and crafts. I bought a new pendulum, got some tea, and pondered what to do next. I was due home in a few hours.

I looked over the available workshops. There was a workshop honoring the Goddess Oshun that looked good, also a fairy ritual designed to raise energy for sex magick—so tempting. Or I could call

Oz. *Could I call Oz?* Oz told me we had clearance to talk, but I felt reticent. I probably shouldn't call him. I needed to prepare to give him up, but—*legally* I could still call Oz.

I grabbed my phone and dialed.

"You rang?" he asked playfully.

"I bought a pendulum at my witch convention."

"Oh yeah?"

"Do you know what a pendulum is?"

"Sure, I know a lot about pendulums," then he paused, his deep baritone laugh coming across the airwaves, "Well, I was going to say, 'A pendulum is a mass at the end of a string whose natural period is 2π times the square root of L over g. Pendulums oscillate back and forth after being exposed to some stimulus. Their purpose is to show Coriolis force and to give college freshmen majoring in physics something to derive.' But since that's nowhere near what you're talking about, I rephrase my response to say, 'I know nothing about pendulums; please educate me.'"

"My pendulum sounds like more fun than your pendulum. My pendulum answers yes or no questions. Can yours do that?"

Just then I was interrupted by friends with whom I was sharing a room, loud and rowdy, fresh from the hot tub. I found a staircase where I had cell reception, then sat down on the cool cement steps. Time flew by as it always did when I was talking with Oz.

We were at least an hour into our discourse when Oz asked, "How many people have you been in love with?"

Who would qualify as someone I had been in love with? There was one instance of puppy love, quite a few great lays, a boyfriend who turned out to be such a resounding disappointment that I would relegate the feelings I had for him as delusional. I described my past amours—high in the sex pleasure arena but low in terms of intimacy and love.

Oz confessed, "It has been so scary for me to be emotionally close to anyone, really. I've only slept with five women, and I was in love with all five."

I found that profoundly sweet—and refreshing after the parade of poly man-hos. Oz explained that he felt vulnerable having sex, that he needed an emotional connection. Oz's vulnerability made him so much more appealing than the sex artists. I imagined that sex with him would have significant meaning. I loved that he could not separate love from sex.

"So, you've had a lot of lovers?" he asked again. "How many times have you been in love?"

Clearly there was only one answer.

"Hank is the only person I've been in love with."

"So, you aren't in love with me?"

I shifted on the cold cement step—the question took me completely by surprise. I hesitated. It was momentous to acknowledge what was happening in such romantic terms—and it was clearly true.

"I am so in love with you," I said.

"I am in love with you, Grace."

We were both silent.

Then Oz went on, "Grace, if we are allowed to be friends, and you meet your sexual partner, if you fall in love, will you take care of me? When you tell me, will you be careful with me?"

"Nobody could ever replace you in my heart. There will never be another Oz. I will always love you no matter who I fall in love with."

Oz was silent.

I sounded like a poly leaflet: "Yes, of course, I'll be careful with you."

"Your second statement has more substance for me than the first. When it happens, you'll be gentle with me?"

"Yes, I'll be gentle." The stairwell suddenly felt cavernous. "Oz, I've been thinking—if we have to say good-bye, can we do it in a session with Lily? I'll need help."

He agreed. We were at a crossroads that would have to be final. We kept talking for hours. I could not hang up; he could not hang up. So we continued talking in the stairwell, as I packed, as I drove home. I pulled up in front of my house and sat in the driver's seat. Hank was inside waiting to celebrate Valentine's Day together. We had presents for each other and then we would take the kids out to our favorite Chinese restaurant.

"I'm having trouble hanging up."

"Let's count to three together—and on three we'll hang up."

"Brilliant!" I said. "One—"

"Wait. Wait one second. Grace, I love you so much."

"I love you too. I love you so much. *Now we must do it.*"

Then we started the countdown again and somehow on three, my finger depressed the red "end" button, which looked glaringly mean. I swung my feet around and placed them on the black asphalt of the street and stood up. I felt a physical jolt that had become familiar. It always accompanied a transition back into my life after saying good-bye to Oz.

That night I woke up at three a.m. In the dark quiet it was clear to me that even if Oz and I were allowed to be friends, it would not be enough. The more contact I had with Oz, the more I wanted him as a lover. I was deeply in love and would never be satisfied with a platonic relationship. My presence was not helping his marriage. *I had to go away.* I e-mailed Oz:

> I think it's best for me to say good-bye. I am too afraid that my presence is creating more pain.

In the morning, Oz called me to say that he had to find a way to "have both of us" in his life. He asked for more time. I felt myself wavering but the truth was, when Oz asked me not to go—*I felt a complete inability to leave.*

But I wasn't sure about Oz. *Couldn't he feel his wife's pain?* It frightened me. But I also empathized with Oz; there seemed to be something vital missing from his marriage.

The next day Oz called to say that there was no chance of our being allowed to be friends. He was now in a position where he had to "pick between us." He also said he was so anxious he'd gotten sick—he had a fever and couldn't eat. He told me he'd lost five pounds. He was burning up inside and staying home sick from his engineering job. He talked primarily about his children. He didn't want to break up his family.

The following day Oz called sounding exhausted.

"Can I ask you something?" he said.

"Sure, you can ask me anything."

Oz groaned. Moments went by.

"If…if…we were lovers, could we—" he started breathing heavily and couldn't go on.

"It's okay. Tell me, you can trust me."

My chest was tightening.

"Could we have unprotected sex?"

"Yes, of course. We can make love skin to skin, nothing in between us."

"Can I ask you something else?" Oz was gaining momentum.

"Yes."

My heart was beating faster, every word felt crucial, a testimony, a pledge.

"Have you gone through menopause?"

Whoa—buy me a drink, Sonny! Sweet-talk me before dropping the conversational bomb!

There was a nine-year age difference between us, Oz being on the sunny side of death. I had thought about this in a whimsical sort of way, priding myself in being a hot cougar. Now I was seeing the downside. Oz was worried that I may be hormonally depleted, a dried-up, shriveled womb that he'd signed on to drive for many years. I staggered a bit but regained my balance.

"No, I haven't gone through menopause. Why do you ask?"

"I am just so afraid, even if I leave Susan, that somehow I'll never get to fully have you, you won't want me, or you'll lose your attraction for me, or I won't get enough of you."

It occurred to me how much he'd be losing to be with me. The stakes were so high for him.

"My love is real, I am fully available to you."

"Do you remember that time outside of Pumping Iron Gym?"

"Yes," I replied.

We had shorthand to describe so many fleeting moments and brief sightings. I remembered *Pumping Iron*. I was coming out from my workout, my muscles twitching, feeling like the great Artemis herself, when I saw Oz's car. I had memorized his license plate. *He was near.* A Pilates studio I had referred him to was close by. I went inside the studio, looking for Oz, even though I was forbidden to see him. My face must have been striking because a trainer friend saw me surveying the studio and asked, "Are you looking for someone?"

"No," I replied feeling slightly mad. I went back out onto the sidewalk.

I checked his meter: fifteen minutes left, a lifetime to wait. My heart pounded. I took out a piece of paper to write a note in my scarlet red lipstick, but my hands shook so badly that I stopped. A gym buddy came outside. His motorcycle was next to Oz's car. We chatted but I could barely hear his words, so consumed was I by the intoxicating thought that at *any moment Oz would step near me*, his body brushing by mine. After several minutes I collected myself. I told my friend I had to go, got into my car, and drove away.

"I saw you from the window. You were talking to that body-builder by my car. I thought, 'That's Grace! Standing by my car! What do I do?' That part of you scares me."

"What do you mean?"

"We had agreed to no contact, and then there you were by my car."

"Do you know how many times I've longed for you in the past three years? Do you know how many times I prayed for an answer, a creative solution? I avoided seeing you not once but hundreds of times. Pumping Iron Gym took me by surprise. Your car appeared out of the blue and it was like bumping into you in Indonesia. It was so unexpected—none of the rules could possibly apply in *Indonesia*!"

"I know, I know," Oz laughed softly.

"This is a crazy-powerful, inconvenient love. You have so much more to lose than I do. If there is any way to make your marriage work, *do it*. But if you choose to be with me, I'll love you like you've never been loved before. I promise you."

The next day Oz asked me to do a session with Lily. Oz included me in a text to her:

> I think everybody is in a state of surrender, waiting for the next step to become clear.

Then Oz texted me privately:

> My primary goal is to understand you so that I can make better decisions about my life. Please help me keep that predominantly in mind.

That day, Hank and I went to get the oil changed in our car. While it was happening I told Hank that there was a possibility Oz would leave his marriage. I asked him if he was with me in this.

Hank said he was. I told Hank about the upcoming counseling session with Oz, and Hank gave me permission to go.

Thirty minutes before the session, my hair, makeup, and outfit were in place. Hank was at a business meeting. I had fed my kids and prepped them on their homework. I paced my living room, waiting. When my babysitter was five minutes late I called her. When she was ten minutes late, I redialed her number and tried to prevent myself from hyperventilating. Fifteen minutes later she called from a session with her jazz band and said she would be there in twenty minutes. *Why were these sixteen-year-old harlots continually foiling me?* I texted her to get over here, pronto! She arrived a few minutes later looking a little scared to be in the same room with me.

I drove to downtown San Francisco, parked my car, and started sprinting down Market Street. I found the turn-of-the-century high-rise that had a bronze plate reading 1904. I rushed inside, hearing the click of my black go-go boots against the gray marble floor of the lobby. I pressed the button for the elevator. *Hurry!* I had called Oz forty-five minutes ago telling him of my predicament. "Just get here" was all he said. Another plaque by the elevator button stated that this building had survived the infamous 1906 San Francisco earthquake. This was the perfect setting for tonight's epic meeting.

I got off the elevator into a long hallway of offices with pebbled glass and large dark-mahogany doors that looked like they'd housed the Pinkerton Detective Agency. I walked quite a ways down the hall, checking the office numbers. Then I heard muffled voices. *Oz's voice.* Although we had been talking all week, I had not seen him in the flesh in nearly half a year.

I knocked lightly. The voices stopped. A second later the door flung open and Oz stood before me, like a Viking, his body tall and lean. I smiled, and then without hesitation he grabbed me and pulled me into his arms, holding me tightly. I was struck by how close and affectionately he held me. After many seconds I disengaged.

We sat down, me on the couch, Oz in an armchair near Lily. We had a quiet moment, which felt momentous.

Oz gazed at me and said, "I'm so happy you're here."

I smiled at him.

I put a pillow in my lap to hide the red velvet minidress I was wearing, which suddenly seemed wildly wrong. Lily gave a speech welcoming us. I could see that even for her the stakes were high; a lot was riding on this meeting. Occasionally she and Oz exchanged glances and referred to moments and realizations in their work together. I looked at Oz while she talked. He was gaunt, his jawline even more pronounced. But there was an appealing spareness to his muscle, like he'd been running a long race and had shed whatever was unnecessary.

After the check-in, Lily asked if I wanted to voice any concerns.

I turned to Oz, "I am afraid that if you come be with me, you'll resent me because I still have Hank."

"Thanks for bringing that up. I have thought about that. Tell me, how would it work between you, me, and Hank?"

The thoughtfulness gave me pause; once again I was reminded of the direness of his situation. He had to choose—there was no gray area for him. We discussed schedules, date nights, and the guidelines Hank, Valerie, and I had created to share each other. Oz nodded ever so slightly. He was very serious, but he did laugh when I said, "I know that if you leave your marriage the shit will hit the fan in our community. If we were on *Oprah*, I'd get stoned."

I concluded with, "But you are worth it. I'll weather any storm to have you."

Oz took a quick intake of breath, his eyes moistened. We looked at each other for several beats.

Oz went on. "Before you arrived, Lily and I were discussing that, for me, this is really a choice between stasis and the growth path. Before I met you I was so dead. I feel like you gave me my life back. I had this stable, secure life, but it had no meaning. You woke me up. You are on a growth path and I need you; I need a life that has you in it."

I smiled at him.

"Do you think Hank would talk to Susan?" Oz asked.

"He would, but only if Susan asked him directly."

Oz nodded solemnly. It was striking to me that even though Oz had to choose, he was still fighting to have both of us. The room was quiet.

Lily said, "You could have done it. You could have loved both these women really well. I have no doubt of that."

A tingling went through my body as I heard her speak in the *past tense*. No one was saying it out loud, but it was clear to me: Oz had made a decision—the die was cast. Whatever happened from this moment forward, there would be no more good-byes between us.

We walked out past the marble lobby and into the cool air of Market Street. Throngs of people surrounded the cable car turntable. There was a street performer riding a unicycle. He had captured the attention of the waiting crowd. Shoppers poured out of the stores. Oz stuffed his hands into the pockets of his jacket. He seemed charged with volts of energy yet also sweetly calm.

"You talk," he said. "I am too happy to speak."

We were walking in sync side by side. I noticed the antique street lamps lining the street. Had they always been this golden? I squinted up at them. Then I looked at the people around us, the headlights of cars, the skyscrapers with their blinking lights—everything was shimmering with a bright amber hue. A feeling was streaming through my veins, an ethereal lightness, as if I were not walking but lightly skimming the edges of the earth. Oz loved me so much he was changing his entire world to be with me. I had done the same to be with him when I opened my marriage. This was a great love.

Oz asked to walk me to my car in the parking garage.

"What time is it?" I asked.

"What day is it?" Oz replied.

We reflected that it had been only ten days since Dark Tuesday, the day I texted Oz that I was at a crossroads. Now we were both at a huge crossroads. When I first texted Oz I was still thinking of myself as possibly nutty. I was failing to create a situation that worked for me. Now I trusted my emotional compass—if I discovered what I needed and followed it with action, miracles could happen. I was sure our love was worth fighting for. I was imagining a life in which I could have Oz and my family. When I thought back to Dark Tuesday, me lying on my bed morose, it felt like a lifetime ago, when it seemed likely I would never have a love life that worked. We commented on how warped it felt that that day had been just over a week ago. Another dilation of time had taken place. Somehow I'd slipped between the worlds, into a different reality and time zone, and here was Oz beside me.

We came to the parking garage, entered the elevator, then disembarked two flights up. We stopped at my car standing across from each other.

"Can I hug you?" I asked.

"Yes."

We embraced. I pulled away to look at his face. Then we hugged again. I nuzzled my head into the crook of his neck. Our breathing started to sync. Then I disengaged, pulling a rose quartz from my pocket.

"I got this stone for you. It will help you."

"I don't need it."

"But it's a talisman; I've charged it with good fortune."

"You are my good fortune."

I smiled, then slid into his arms. We held each other a moment longer before parting.

Chapter 11

The morning after our session with Lily was Merlin's fifth birthday party. Oz asked in a text if he and his son, Liam, could come to the party. Oz had not stepped foot in my home for two and half years, yet we traipsed through my house, passing each other on the stairs as we were marauded by Merlin, Liam, and a dozen other kids playing tag. Our eyes would meet and we'd grin as we were pushed forward by the unruly band of five-year-olds. At one point we found each other elbow to elbow in a quiet corner.

"How is it going?" I asked.

"We are at a standoff," Oz said.

After the party, I crawled into bed—exhausted and buzzed. I'd been averaging three maybe four hours of sleep a night for the past week. I could hardly eat. I felt a little like I was hovering above my body—ungrounded and watching myself as if I were in a dream. I fell into a deep sleep, and when I awoke two hours later the house was quiet. I reached for my cell phone. Oz had texted me two words:

Call me.

I dialed his number. He picked up.

"We have decided to divorce." His voice was tired, somber.

"I am so sorry."

I felt sad for him, and awkward. I sat quietly, not knowing how to comfort him.

"Will you spend the night with me?" Oz asked.

"Yes."

We decided to meet in two hours. I'd dreamed for years about a date with Oz—now here it was. I was consumed with an all-encompassing urgency to get on that date—*now!* If I had stopped to contemplate why—which I did not as I ran around getting ready—it would have made sense. For years, Oz and I had given each other up repeatedly. Now I was elated on the surface, but it still seemed that at any moment the hand of fate could pull him away from me. I felt an urgency to act quickly. Two hours later, I paced the living room waiting for Oz's arrival. *When was Oz coming? I couldn't hang on another second!* Oz texted me that he was on some "special mission."

Finally the doorbell rang and there stood Oz with a dozen roses in his hands. He stepped inside. I shut the vestibule door and turned to take him upstairs to say a quick good-bye to Hank.

"Hey, hold on a second."

Oz pulled me close, his body fitting perfectly against mine. He leaned down and in an instant the long-anticipated kiss was done. Our bodies fused for a moment.

"Thanks for the flowers," I smiled. "What a nice thing to do."

"I am a nice guy," Oz said plaintively, and it occurred to me how maligned he must feel at this moment, choosing to leave his wife.

"Come upstairs and say good-bye to Hank and Valerie."

Valerie and Hank were seated in the sunroom. The kids were in our bedroom watching a movie. When Oz and I walked in, Hank stood up, rather stiffly. He nodded at Oz. There was tension in the air, but at the time I barely noticed it. In the last twenty-four hours I had been updating Hank about Oz. An hour ago I had texted Hank that I was going out with Oz. It was my date night. It didn't occur to me to get permission to spend the night with Oz. After all, Hank had spent many nights with Valerie while I sat home, the jolly poly good sport.

"So you two will take care of each other while we are gone?" I asked somewhat facetiously. Yet, somewhere in my being I knew Hank needed to be taken care of at this moment. Nevertheless, I was entrusting him to Valerie.

Valerie quickly glanced at Hank, who looked blank. I saw a look pass between them, but I was almost stoned with the adrenal rush to be off with Oz, so much so that I didn't for a second consider I might be shirking some other responsibility.

Right now—*I had to leave.* Every second felt like a bomb ticking, and I needed to get out into the sweet cool night. In the conscious part of my mind this was all just polite protocol. Hank and Valerie were in love, and I had given them my blessing. Why shouldn't I expect the same? How was this any different from what Hank had been doing for the last several months? But deep down I knew what was happening for me was very different in Hank's mind. I was to find out later just how radically differently Hank saw this moment. But at this point in time, if anyone had jumped in front of the door, I would have told him to step away from the exit and then bit him hard if he didn't move—and move fast. It was my turn now. *My turn—and I'd been waiting years to take my turn.* Wild horses couldn't have slowed me down.

Oz and I said our good-byes and walked to the car; I was carrying my 1950s makeup case, with white leather trim. It was the perfect miniature overnight bag. It contained lube, sex toys, fresh panties, and a toothbrush—all a girl needed for an amorous night.

"What's that?" Oz said, as I placed the makeup case on his backseat.

"Oh, that's my overnight bag."

"Are we going to be together overnight?"

Oz looked surprised. When he asked me to spend the night with him I naturally assumed we'd rent a hotel room. Not necessarily have sex—it occurred to me that we had been occupying vastly different worlds in the last six months. But I honestly didn't care what we did; I was just excited to be together, and if we talked all night that would be splendid.

I shrugged, "If we aren't spending the night together, I guess I overpacked."

We sat in the silver Fiat.

"I feel like I'm sixteen," Oz said, "and just got approved by your mom and dad."

I giggled. "It was a bit awkward, huh?"

"Where shall we go?"

I didn't care, so Oz picked his favorite vegetarian restaurant and we were off. We parked and meandered down the sidewalk to the restaurant. It was nightfall and the darkness enveloped us. Oz stopped, pulled me close, then leaned my body back, kissing me, our second kiss. We knew each other so well, trusted each other so much, loved each other, but we didn't know each other's bodies. As we walked he kept me near him. His touch was affectionate, which struck me because he had been so stiff and reserved for so long. I wasn't sure if that had been the situation or his personality. I was seeing a new side to him. It felt new yet oddly familiar to embrace.

At the restaurant, I watched Oz as he studied the menu. There were lights hanging over the table like glass cocoons radiating soft light. I could hear the clatter from the kitchen as the staff rushed to prepare food. A Saturday-night crowd was at the brown-speckled marble bar sipping fuchsia-colored drinks in long-stemmed martini glasses. *We were having dinner together.* I'd had dreams about this moment, brief images of us holding hands, arms stretching across the vast tabletop. Oz put down his menu. I had a plan ready to get through any initial awkwardness.

"I'll set the timer on my cell phone for thirty minutes and tell you all the things I love about you," I suggested.

Oz smiled wearily. "I think I just want to talk. Could we just talk?"

"Of course."

It surprised me a bit that he didn't want all the focus on him, but I liked that instead a reciprocal conversation would do. It made me realize that we still had so much to know about each other.

"Perhaps we could do that mirroring exercise? The one in the book you recommended."

"Alright," I said.

"I feel so exhausted and burned out. I tried so many ways to make it work."

I mirrored his words. Oz had been working on his marriage for two years. It was still a mystery to me what was not working. I felt sad for him, but I couldn't deny that I was happy to be sitting with him, even though I knew that he had paid a much higher price to be here tonight.

Oz asked if I wanted to be mirrored. I declined. The contrast in our emotional spaces was so extreme that I felt self-conscious. He seemed to be experiencing the end of a long attempt to create a marriage in which he could both evolve and keep his family intact. For both Oz and me this was the most compelling reason to do poly—to keep our families together. The idea that you could keep your family and get to add in a new person was radically thrilling, and, for me, it seemed like it might be possible. But tonight it was clear it wasn't going to work out for Oz. I felt how somber the situation was for him but at the same time there was tremendous happiness that we were together. I put my hand across the table and we brushed fingertips.

"You forgot to mirror the most important part," Oz said.

"What's that?" I asked.

"Grace, I love you so much. I had to have you no matter how big the price."

I clasped his hand, lacing my fingers between his. I slid over to his side of the table and onto the padded booth. His huge hand engulfed my palm. I leaned into his torso, tucking my shoulder under his arm.

"I am so exhausted. I just want to go to a hotel," Oz said. "We could lie on the bed and check out each other's naked bodies…"

"That sounds great."

Thirty minutes later we stood across from the concierge at a hotel just off the bay. Oz pulled out a pile of credit and debit cards, with his license on top, all secured with a large metal binder clip—very utilitarian and functional. He glided a card across the counter to the hotel clerk. I stood by his side observing while he signed the credit card slip. Normally in these dating situations I'd have pulled out my wallet and paid half, the poly credo when dating. Could a guy with five girlfriends be expected to pay for every hotel room? But at the restaurant when I reached for my wallet, Oz said quietly, "What are you doing?"

"Well, I am paying for my part of the bill." My voice had wavered. I was the good, if slightly financially burdened, feminist.

"Put your money away," Oz had said softly.

We waited while the concierge got us a room key. I studied Oz, fascinated to see him moving through the mundane world. I still didn't know the most basic facts about him. What was his morning liquid of choice? Tea, coffee, orange juice? He stood waiting. Out of the corner of his eye, he noticed me watching him. Without pretense he smiled at me like an unabashed sixth-grader—shy, unsure, but friendly. My eyes perused his body again. I liked his packaging. He wore dark jeans that were snug around his muscular legs and slim hips. His pin-striped shirt was buttoned to the neck. I could see the outline of his biceps, but still there was something restrained about him—the professorial librarian.

We opened the door to the room. Oz excused himself and went to the bathroom. I walked to the window. I felt buzzed but oddly relaxed. I looked out onto the parking lot. This wasn't a room with a bay view, but who cared about gazing at the bay? Across from me in the hills there were thousands of lights shimmering from homes tucked up on the ridge.

Oz came up behind me and wrapped his arms around my waist. I started to turn toward him, but he stopped me.

"No, stand still," he undid my belt buckle. "This is a very sexy belt. I've seen you wear it many times." He kissed my neck, "Now I get to take it off you."

"You like my belt?" I whispered breathlessly.

I had bought this belt thinking of Oz seeing me wear it. It was retro 1960s with a big circular buckle, something Janis Joplin might wear around her hip huggers. I'd worn it with bell-bottom jeans, my uniform many a day dropping off my kids at school. It tickled me that Oz had noticed it.

Oz was bending my body slightly, holding me tightly to him. I gasped a little as he unlatched the belt. *Where was the librarian?* Oz's relaxed sexual prowess was unexpected. After removing my jeans, he peeled off my red cotton T-shirt, then pulled me backward against his chest, reaching for my breasts, pressing his lips against my neck.

He was clearly going to drive. I was a bit amazed. Oz had seemed like a shy little boy when sex came up in conversation. I had expected I might have to coax him along. But Oz commandeered me toward the bed, then pressed me down on the paisley duvet, kissing me urgently. Then he stopped, perched on his elbows above me.

"Be right back," he announced and leaped off the bed and went into the bathroom. *What would happen next?*

He returned a moment later holding floss between his two index fingers and thumbs; he stood diligently flossing between each molar.

"Flossing?" I asked him, but somehow it didn't surprise me.

This was more what I expected of Oz: the repressed geek, the flossing nerd. Oz explained that he had skipped dentist visits for five years, which resulted in a root canal—thus he had become a flossing devotee.

As he told me this story he stood in a rose-colored silk thong, clearly oblivious to the striking picture he created, almost as if his physicality was inconsequential. But it wasn't inconsequential to me. I was having a hard time regulating my breathing. The silk thong housed his more-than-generous member. I was fascinated by his nonchalance.

"I like your thong," I said.

Oz was oblivious. Any other man would have been aware of the spectacle he created. Oz looked like a poster you'd see in the Castro District. He finished flossing, then jumped onto the bed next to me.

"Thank you. I ordered several of them. I wanted to learn to be gentler with myself. Silk is soft and gentle."

"You ordered pink silk thongs to get in touch with your feminine side?"

"Yes, you could say it like that. I was trying to develop that side of me."

I grinned.

"What?" Oz started laughing too.

"Nothing. I like how you decided to grow parts of yourself."

"You were my inspiration. I couldn't have you, so I had to learn to nurture myself."

Oz crawled closer, wrapping his arms around me, his body feeling weighty. I liked his style, sweet and vulnerable but in charge too. He pinned me to the bed. I immediately got wet by how much stronger he was than I. Oz unclasped my bra, then removed my panties. We were now fully undressed. Oz explored me with his hands and mouth. There were so many times I could remember him near me, looking at his body but adhering to the invisible boundary between us, which was like the thick Plexiglas surrounding a bank teller that prevents you from grabbing some cash. Now, all boundaries were gone.

Oz stopped suddenly and sat up, "I want to turn on more lights so I can look at you."

I preferred soft lighting, but Oz flipped on the large bedside lamp. He sat on his heels gazing at me without any pretense, hungrily, viscerally taking me in.

"You are the most beautiful woman I've ever slept with," he breathed.

I felt a ripple of delight at the sentiment. Then he was on top of me again, grabbing a fistful of my hair, pulling my head back, and entering me. He was so free, aggressively taking what he needed from me. I was somewhat astonished but—I loved it. After lovemaking, Oz rolled over on his side, and propped his head up with one hand.

"Is there a place on your body that you feel is ugly?"

"What?"

"You said once that you had body-image issues. Is there a place you feel isn't beautiful?"

I was usually the one putting Oz under the microscope. I hedged. The truth was I wasn't eager to retread over this well-worn territory. I loved my body but often I'd catch myself looking in the mirror like a cop frisking a criminal, brusque and suspicious.

"I strive to love all parts of my body." I said.

Oz's eyes warmed when he said gently, "That's nice. Can we try again? Where do you feel ugly?"

Damn, he didn't buy my New Age spiel. I paused, internally cornered. I hated to point out my physical flaws—it went against my grain. But there was a bigger issue. I knew that disowned feelings showed up in the body; I saw this again and again with my clients and myself. And the primary place my disowned feelings showed up was in my ass. I had always enjoyed robust health, but if anything went wrong, it manifested in the small Bermuda triangle of my butt. But I couldn't imagine revealing the history of my sorry ass to O.

Oz was waiting.

I said quietly, "I have a little cellulite situation on my ass."

Oz turned me against his chest, spooning me. I could feel him moving down my back, planting kisses as he traveled. He got to my ass and softly brushed it with his lips. I felt exposed, emotionally nude and wildly vulnerable. Like a deer poised to bolt, my muscles tightened. Oz gently caressed my body. I felt a knot deep in my gut undo itself. I was stunned realizing quite suddenly, that this—*right here, right now*—was what I had wanted for so long: fantastic sex, aggressive, lusty sex, and with a man I unequivocally loved. Getting it almost made me feel transported, delivered to a new universe. At that moment, I knew even if Hank asked me to, I could never let Oz go.

The next afternoon I beelined to Good Vibrations, a sex shop famous for its sex-positive atmosphere and mostly female staff. I was looking for equipment to tone my pelvic floor. At the end of our lovemaking, Oz had casually asked, "Do you do Kegels?" I had answered yes, after all, Pilates was one giant Kegel. When I asked him why he brought it up, he replied, "No reason."

The conversation did not sit well with me. I found a pair of Ben Wa balls, small stainless-steel balls you hold in your vagina by doing one constant Kegel. I stood before an entire shelf of them, determined to pick the ones that would tone my pussy to such maximum strength that if Oz got his cock within inches of me, the muscles of my pelvic floor would suck his dick up to my navel.

At that moment Oz called me. I told him where I was. Oddly enough, he was right around the corner. We had parted just hours prior and had both gone off to be with our children. Hank and I had made pancakes with Tallulah and Merlin. After breakfast and a trip to the library, I'd stepped out to get groceries, and then rushed to the sex store to get tools for my sagging pussy. Oz told me he'd come meet me at the store. I hung up and perused the balls. Oz walked in. He adjusted his yellow slicker, shaking off the rain. It still felt miraculous to be in the same room. He inquired what I was up to. I explained.

"Wow," Oz said, after I described the upcoming dangers of my soon-to-be maximally toned Grade-A pussy, "I am going to have to recalibrate my pleasure meters."

"Recalibrate your pleasure meters? I love how you talk. Explain."

"Well, the pleasure meters in my life were in this range—" he fanned his figures over a 45-degree span.

"So your meter went to, say, zero to thirty."

"Yes. Right. Now with you it tops out at, say, sixty—"

"Let's say one hundred, why not one hundred?" I added. *Why not get a top score if you could?*

Just then Hank texted me that I needed to get home *now*. I rushed back, where the pleasure meters were distinctly lower. The house was quiet when I arrived. Hank and the kids were upstairs. I figured I'd earn some brownie points by cleaning up the kitchen. After a few minutes, Hank walked down the stairs. He leaned on the counter watching me cleaning.

"I got some salmon for dinner," I announced. "and a bottle of Chardonnay."

"Valerie is very upset."

"Why?"

"Did you read her e-mail?"

"No, I haven't checked my e-mails today."

He opened his cell phone and handed it to me. There was a very long e-mail addressed to me and Oz (with Hank cc'd), but it was mostly directed at me. I read it quietly. Valerie thought Oz and I were "not doing poly." And she felt that I used her to take emotional care of Hank while I went off with Oz.

"Yikes," I mumbled. I felt queasy. I looked at Hank, whose face was blank, unreadable. "Are you upset too?"

Hank pulled up a chair at the counter. There was a long silence. I suddenly flashed on the first month Hank and Valerie were together. At that time I couldn't imagine the bliss he must have been feeling having me, the kids, our lovely home, *and* a new lover.

I said just that to him. "Aren't you just blissed out? Isn't this a dream come true?" I added.

He shrugged, "Kind of."

"What do you mean?" I asked incredulous. Hank was always downplaying joy.

"It's not all it's cracked up to be. With poly it seems like there's always someone a little pissed off at you."

Now I understood. I wanted Hank to be happy for me. I had been so happy for him, as in some ways his falling in love with Valerie had been a rebirth of our love. I felt so close to him, so thrilled to see him that alive. But I also remembered my adjustment period when he was first with Valerie and I told him we were "officially in crisis." At times, I'd felt territorial or hurt, but I had worked at moving through those feelings. Hank, in contrast, seemed so stony. Couldn't he work with me too? I thought about what the books said about "new relationship energy" and how your partner had to adjust to the new person in your life. Hank interrupted my thoughts.

"I can't believe you spent the night with Oz. We didn't discuss that."

"What…?" I was shocked.

"You didn't talk to me. You just went off with Oz."

I continued haltingly, "But we talked about me being with Oz while we were getting the oil changed in the car." My hands were shaking as I leaned on the counter.

"I said yes to you doing a therapy session with him. I didn't say you could sleep with Oz."

I thought back to the day I asked Hank to get the oil changed in our Jeep. We had sat on a wooden bench waiting for the car. It was a brief but important talk.

I had said, "Oz is doing four sessions with Lily. He wants me to go to the first session. Can I go?"

"Yes," Hank had replied.

"If Oz leaves his marriage, are you with me on this?"

Hank had replied, "Yes."

Hank had always been a man of few words. His "yes" was enough for me to proceed. But Hank remembered this conversation very differently, saying repeatedly that he had said yes only to the counseling session.

We needed help badly. We were in the confusing quagmire of polyamory. In the multiple-relationship scenario there were so many unforeseen events, so many hairpin turns that came at you so fast that you were likely to spin out of control. We were spinning a bit, but I had my hands on the steering wheel trying to steady our drive. The poly books advised that you have a friend or counselor help sort things out. I remembered that Aurora, the leader of my poly support group, was studying to be a therapist. I called her and asked if she'd meet with us.

After dinner, I reread Valerie's e-mail in a stunned stupor. Then I called Oz and we softly discussed what we dubbed the "poly police." I felt smarted by the unfairness.

"Is it poly if you leave your wife?" I asked.

"So there's only one way to do it? And we aren't doing it that one way?" Oz queried.

He was more disturbed to hear about Hank. Oz was scared that Hank would say we couldn't see each other and that I would acquiesce. Oz volunteered to talk to Valerie on the phone and explain himself.

A few days later, Hank and I met Aurora at Cyclops Cave to sort out the mess. We both ran through our scenarios. We were very polarized. Aurora listened quietly. I tried to get Hank to remember our conversation when our car was getting an oil change.

"Remember I said, 'Are you with me if Oz leaves his wife?'"

Hank said, "I thought you meant being friends. I agreed to the sessions, not to you dating Oz."

I was annoyed but too scared to show it. We went back and forth about how I left that night. Hank felt he never got the opportunity to say no. Although Hank didn't say it out loud, what was clear to me was that this was about my being in love with Oz. Being in love was one of those ambiguous subjects in poly conversations that we had never been crystal clear about. But then again, I had been complaining for months about my shallow dating experiences with the poly man-hos. I had clearly wanted more depth and spoke to Hank about it. This all felt like a double standard. After all, Hank was in love with Valerie.

Aurora asked, "Grace, the night you and Oz got together, did you feel that you had been waiting so long and followed everyone's rules and you just had to act now?"

"*Yes!*" I said, thrilled that someone understood me.

"There's how we want to do poly, how we intend to do it, following every bylaw; but sometimes we are ruled by our emotions, and it is an emotional experience to be doing poly."

Then we reviewed the oil-changing conversation yet again. By now I was frustrated by the semantics.

Finally Aurora said, "The only advice I can offer is, never get your oil changed at that place again."

What I took from the conversation was that I was skating on thin ice and that Hank could only handle doing poly when I was with a lover I wasn't enthused about. This did not bode well. I was angry, but overall I was scared. This was going to go awry if Hank could not be generous with me. Perhaps I was swept away by my emotions on the night Oz and I left together. But if Hank had tried to prevent me from choosing Oz as a lover—I wasn't sure what I would have done.

I had read about poly couples who had agreements in which they could deny their partners contact with a particular lover. Others accepted that this came with the turf—one day your partner may date someone you don't want him or her to date. I now understood the deep complexities of both agreements. Hank and I had never directly discussed either of us having the power to demand the other forfeit a potential lover. I had hoped that Hank would grant me the freedom I had granted him.

I went home and called Oz. He was relieved to hear that Hank had not demanded I end the relationship with him. He told me about his call with Valerie. Valerie had assumed that he had abruptly left his wife. Oz had explained to her, patient on the surface but insulted internally, how much effort he had invested over many years to try to make his marriage work.

In the next few weeks we were to find that this was a common assumption: Oz was the bad guy. He had left his wife for his Pilates instructor—to do poly. He was a screwball. We laughed at the cliché, but over time we were to discover how serious the ramifications of this bigotry could be.

After our session with Aurora, Hank and I were in a careful truce on the subject of what had happened. We did not agree. But Hank allowed me to continue dating Oz. Hank was in a period of adjustment. A few days after Hank and I met with Aurora, Oz and I had our second date. Oz picked me up and we drove to Robert Sibley Volcanic Regional Preserve, home to dormant volcanoes. We climbed a steep hill covered with a thicket of trees. It was green and lush, with a slight mist from an earlier shower. But at the crest of the hill the sun shone brightly, and we were treated to spectacular views of the mountains and the city in the distance. Oz pulled off my cotton T-shirt and skirt, then placed me on the moss. He removed his shirt and crouched above me, biting my nipples, then entering me. After making love, Oz jumped up like an energized teenage boy, insisting on taking my picture. But when he pulled out his cell phone he stood transfixed for a moment. "Grace, you are incredibly lovely." He looked striking standing above me. I felt like Morgaine from *The Mists of Avalon*, the Queen of the Fairies with her Pagan Prince.

Oz snapped the picture, then turned his cell phone toward me, displaying the photo of me laying serenely on the velvety moss. I warned him it better not end up on some geeky site for computer nerds who have a fetish for outdoor sex. He assured me it would not. Then I got my cell phone and took a picture of Oz. Later, over drinks at a bar overlooking the city, I gasped when I pulled up the photo. He stood staring down at me, fully erect with a bold smile on his lips, a god of the wilderness. We sat looking over the bay, me sipping a Chardonnay, Oz drinking a mint julep.

"I looked at your OkCupid page," Oz said.

"Oh yeah?"

"Those pictures of you are really hot," he started. "But everything feels so unstable. I just left my wife. It feels so precarious with Hank. I don't want you to date. Will you take down your page?"

Oz's face looked tight with anxiety. I was amazed again by how quickly circumstances changed in the world of polyamory. I found myself doing a quick inventory of my priorities. What was most important right now was integrating Oz into my life while maintaining my love with Hank. I was already experiencing what a potentially major feat this would be. I thought about Bobby Z. Our relationship was so new—I figured he'd be okay with the breakup.

Oz's cell rang. It was his mother. I fingered my cell phone and picked it up. I went to my OkCupid page and opened my inbox. It was packed with a lovely onslaught of e-mails from man-sluts from San Francisco to Nova Scotia to Tel Aviv—some in their twenties imploring *me* not to be *ageist* (!) and give them a chance. Their messages were like a box of delectable candies, sweet but not filling. There was a new note from Bobby Z. I winced as I read his kind words.

I looked over at Oz chatting up his mom.

Oz cupped the phone, "My mother wants you to come visit her."

I nodded and gave the thumbs-up. Hank, the kids, and I were heading to Boston the next month for Passover; I'd make a plan to have lunch with her. I looked down again at my OkCupid profile. My eye caught upon a new message from a twentysomething in San Francisco:

I'm not even going to pretend that we're a good match, but oh-my-god are you gorgeous! OK, I feel much better now... ;)

Mrs. Robinson lives on. *This was some good smack.*

This chapter of poly had been an incredible adventure. Opening my marriage and getting to date men who were excited to know me had been titillating and a healing salve to my bruised ego after Hank's pillow barricades. Now I was in a new stage of the odyssey and the stakes were higher. Oz was the exceptional and rare lover I'd longed for, and his feelings were a priority. I wanted to respond to them as we moved forward. His position was far more precarious than mine. I decided to focus on building our relationship and making Oz feel secure in my love.

The next day I called Bobby Z. I thought it would be a brief but meaningful good-bye, so I was shocked when he was truly pained. I expected it to be an easy bounce for the guy—he had two other girlfriends, after all. But Bobby Z explained in slowly measured words what he deemed one of the hardest aspects of the poly lifestyle: the good-byes. He proved himself to be a true class act, sending me flowers that afternoon and offering his timeshare in Santa Cruz if Oz and I wanted a night away. If this was how poly people broke up, I was more than impressed.

A few days later I met Oz at his new apartment near the Berkeley Marina for our third date. With penthouse views of San Francisco and the Golden Gate Bridge as our background, we immediately starting kissing and caressing each other on the couch. But I interrupted to tell Oz about breaking up with Bobby Z. This news seemed to embolden Oz's affections. But when I told him about Bobby Z's offer of the timeshare, he growled at the idea. Oz was clearly jealous—which, frankly, I was fine with—even though it was the forbidden poly emotion. I wanted time to build our relationship; his jealousy seemed to signify the same desire.

"Oh, baby," I said as I put his hand on my pussy. "Are you a little jealous?"

He answered by picking me up, carrying me to the bed, undoing his belt, and entering me. After making love we continued our conversation. Then Oz asked about Hank.

I replied that things were good. But, in actuality, they were tense.

Just that afternoon Hank had said, "I don't want you to do sleepovers with Oz. He left his wife. He can't have mine." I was racing with cortisol as we sat at the kitchen table talking. He cut back on sleepovers with Valerie because of the exhaustion factor. It was too hard to be back in the saddle flipping pancakes for the kids the next day. For the past several weeks he'd slept over at Valerie's only occasionally on weekends.

This also allowed us to maintain the façade of being "out with friends" with our kids. Our agreement was to absolutely be back in bed by five a.m., when the kids were beginning to stir. But after just one school-night sleepover, I understood why Hank only did sleepovers on special occasions. I'm a girl who loves nine hours of downtime, so it had been brutal to get up and put in a full day on just five hours of sleep. Still, it was unfair that he got to decide when we had this privilege. But I wasn't going to argue; I could fall through the thin ice at any moment.

I dreaded telling Oz about this new agreement with Hank. Hank had granted me one more night with Oz. In a way, I was okay with sleeping at home near my kids, but I knew the power dynamics would freak Oz out. I resolved to tell Oz in the morning about Hank's decision. Poly had sounded so straightforward in all the books. But now I realized that reading little vignettes of perfect poly scenarios was not the same as living them. The books were like watching a scary movie without the soundtrack. Someone taking an ax in the gut looked banal without the screams of horror. Now that I was dealing with the screams of horror and the full emotional spectrum, it was overwhelming—but worth it to have Oz.

In the morning Oz showered while I got dressed.

We got breakfast at a café near the marina. The sweet fragrance of nearby evening primrose blossoms filled the air—it was finally spring. I got coffee and a cranberry bran muffin. Oz ordered a bagel with cream cheese, with cucumber and tomato on top. I could hardly eat. Since we started our romance I hadn't slept much either. I still felt like I was orbiting Earth, so high to finally have Oz. But the adrenalin I was feeling was more euphoria than fear. Oz looked at my half-eaten muffin.

"May I?" he asked.

"Finish it. I'm done."

He touched what was left of the muffin top, then looked at me. I started formulating a good opener for the bad news. "*Oz, we need to talk*—"

"I shouldn't eat the crispy part, should I?"

"Help yourself."

He took some muffin into his mouth, and then reached for more. He stopped pensively, holding a cranberry between his thumb and index finger, then met my gaze.

"These red berries take me back to your nipples last night."

I bit my lip.

He looked so irresistible eating the muffin and talking about my nipples that I just couldn't bear to bring up Hank's new rule and shatter the bliss. Every moment with Oz felt embossed in gold—I wanted to preserve it. It felt dreamlike. In fact that night I had a dream that captured all I was feeling.

Someone had built the Taj Mahal in my backyard. Breathless, I entered the palace, moving from room to room, my fingertips tracing the magnificent white marble. But it was the feeling of indescribable wonder that I most remember. The same feeling I had when I saw Oz's name in my cell phone "favorites," as awe provoking as watching the moonlight shimmer off the arches and domes of the palace—this blessing—*I have Oz.*

Chapter 12

Hank and I were sitting at our egg-shaped dining table with Aurora, having another therapy session. I had asked Hank if we could discuss the sleepover issue with our therapist. The room had the tension of two countries negotiating a delicate treaty.

Hank stated flatly, "I still don't want you to do sleepovers. You can have your dates but no sleepovers."

I knew this was unfair and illogical. Hank was in love with Valerie and had slept over at her house plenty of times. Why shouldn't I get the same? But it was clear to me that Hank was alarmed by my powerful feelings for Oz. This was not the land of logic. We had not made specific rules about whether we could be in love—and my love for Oz was clearly a threat for Hank.

Aurora listened quietly, and then asserted that a new relationship typically included a rocky adjustment period, and that now Hank was the one adjusting. Deep in my gut I knew that this would be harder for him. Oddly, even though I had accepted the role of the identified wacko, somewhere in time I knew I had become stronger than Hank. He had less internal and external resources to work with. As a wacko, I had a large support system of friends, therapists, and internal tools. Because Hank had played it tough, going it alone for many years, he was going to require a longer adjustment period.

Hank went on, "I don't want to have a beer with Oz."

Oz had e-mailed Hank. He had had the enthusiasm of a second-grader trying to make pals on the first day of school.

"I feel humiliated by this situation and I don't want to be hanging out with Oz."

"I think that's a good choice," said Aurora. "Don't get together with Oz till you feel more secure. Let's focus on your relationship with Grace."

I was grateful Hank was open to my seeing Oz—especially since he was revealing that he felt humiliated. Hank was being generous—in the scope of what he had to give at this time. I knew from experience not to push Hank; if hurt he would retreat further. If this was going to work, I had to put aside any idea of things moving at my pace. We had to go at his pace.

The prickly nature of Hank's jealousy unnerved me. But I desperately wanted to put him at ease while at the same time try to empathize with what he was feeling. I wasn't intimidated by Hank falling in love with Valerie, but I was realizing that I had hoped his falling in love with her would make it easier for him to accept my being in love with Oz. I tried to remember an instance when I felt that threatened by Hank's actions.

His ex-girlfriend Tatiana popped into my head. In our second year together after moving to San Francisco, Hank had reconnected with her. He asked for my permission to take a walk with her in the hills. We had agreed he'd return in the early afternoon. By four o'clock I was deflated, and by five-thirty I was comatose on the couch.

When Hank finally came home, I could hardly speak. He sat me up and made me tea. His face filled with alarm. I couldn't even ask him if they had touched each other. I knew they had, but I also knew that hearing him say it out loud would demolish me. It was too catastrophic to think that Hank could be a male brute ruled by his sexuality. Technically his transgression did fall into our "don't ask, don't tell policy" in effect at the time; but the truth Hank and I learned, but did not speak of that afternoon, was that any infraction of his devotion—physical or otherwise—was too painful. This was a time when I had been so much more fragile than Hank. The memory of his kindness that day made me feel even more loyal to him.

Every several years Tatiana would pop up. She started attending my theater productions, and I grew to rather like her. She reminded me of myself, a seeker, trying to make it right inside herself. Once, when Hank and I had been together for at least fifteen years, I asked him directly if he and Tatiana ever made out. He confessed that they had occasionally kissed, but it had stopped years ago by her request. Oddly, it didn't upset me at all to hear this. Most likely the spaces between her appearances, in which Hank proved again and again to be steadfast and dependable to me, allowed me to titrate slowly into my psyche the contrasting knowledge that Hank might be a bit of a sex dog.

My thoughts were interrupted by Aurora.

"When was the last time you spent quality time together on a date being intimate sexually and emotionally?"

"It's been a while. But I'd like to connect and be sexual again," I offered.

Aurora asked us about our sex life. She concluded, "It seems like one of the reasons you opened up your marriage was because you weren't having enough sex. Your new partner shouldn't be about fulfilling needs that your husband does not. He or she should be like a good tennis partner that plays a slightly different brand of tennis than your spouse plays. I am not sure you two are really poly. True poly isn't about getting something your partner isn't giving."

Now I was beginning to feel annoyed. I needed help beyond terminology. Although I liked Aurora, I had begun to step back from all the "poly experts." It seemed that everyone doing poly had their own unique definition of this concept. Even Newt Gingrich thought he could just inform his wife that he had "opened their marriage." Save Newt's, I respected people's unique styles of poly. It would be better if Hank and I had more sex—but that just wasn't happening. As far as I was concerned, we had set up a situation that incorporated a lot of the polyamorous principles. We were literally "loving many," as the word connotes.

I wanted help with "sharing people" and creating a family, together, in which each of us thrived. That Aurora was mainly focusing on reviving our sex life was irksome. Although I didn't realize it at the time, this began a defining change in my thinking. I needed a broader perspective on our situation and someone with keen insights as to how to make it work—not an attempt to make us poly by her definition of poly. I didn't care what we called our setup—but I wanted a situation in which people were emotionally responsive to each other and our sexuality was understood to be on a spectrum, not a locked static state.

But at the time, I was still compelled to do poly "right" (by Aurora's definition). So a few days later, I made another attempt to reignite my sex life with Hank. I'd coiffed, brushed my teeth, gargled with industrial-strength Listerine, and lay next to Hank in bed. We were kissing, but it wasn't flying.

Hank said, "I need to feel connected to make love."

That was an unexpected low blow. I felt emotionally connected to him, in spite of our sexual disconnect.

"I feel like I'm cheating on Valerie," he informed me again. And then he said with exasperation, "What do you want from me?!"

I looked up at the ceiling, limp with exhaustion and mildly aware of something churning in my gut. Everything I was feeling was crusted over by a primal fear of getting abandoned by Hank, and underneath a quiet flow of lava was seething. *I have done everything possible to connect with you, and I am so done being rejected sexually.* I felt a widening gap in my chest that I could see Hank would never fill.

Sex between Hank and me wasn't working. It was clear to me: following someone else's relationship doctrine, whether "married and monogamous" or "poly and multipartnered" or something else, was not the way through. If the poly ideal was that I play tennis with both the men in my life—so be it. What had originally drawn me to poly was not more rules but the whole idea of thinking out of the relationship box.

When I got out of bed twenty frustrating minutes later, I decided that that was the last and final time I would attempt to seduce Hank. This was the moment when I stepped out of the poly box, as well as the marriage box, and decided to be guided by my own intuition. I would set up situations and agreements born out of what we all needed, not some external doctrine. I didn't care what we called it or who approved. *Fuck it. I am going completely rogue and making my own rules.*

I stood in front of my vanity mirror. It was my big Saturday-night date with Oz. I pulled my red ruched sheath dress past my hips, over breasts, knotting the ties around my neck. My cell phone trilled with Oz's special ring tone that sounded like chapel bells. Oz was texting about our theater tickets. I texted him back that I'd found an interesting play at the Magic Theatre.

At the Magic we sat side by side. I was completely distracted by Oz, who kept staring at me then sliding his hand up my thighs.

"Watch the show," I'd mouth, then smile at him.

After the show we walked down the empty pier to look across the bay at Alcatraz Island. Oz came up behind me, wrapped his arms around my waist, pulling me close. I leaned into him.

"I want you," he whispered.

"So take me."

I put one foot up on the wooden slats of the fence then arched my back. I hiked my dress up, displaying myself to Oz, who gasped with delight. I was readily available, not even wearing a thong— Goddess forbid a panty line. Oz approached every sexual encounter urgently—he grasped my hips, entering me, and I moaned with each thrust. Then the lights went on in the loft above us. We leaped to cover ourselves and ran quickly up the pier giggling.

Back at Oz's apartment we made love again. Oz asked me if I could bike the next morning, and I remembered the bad news.

"Well, actually, I wanted to tell you earlier."

"What?" Oz looked pale.

"Hank says he doesn't want me sleeping over for a while."

"What? Why?"

Should I tell him Hank's stern line—"Oz just left his wife, he isn't getting mine"? *No, that would really shake him up.*

"He's having a hard time adjusting to us," I felt compelled to rush.

Oz's face looked troubled. I could feel him softening inside me.

"It'll be okay."

But when Oz walked me to my car, we stood for several minutes holding each other, me murmuring reassurance.

The next day I managed on a technicality to meet Oz on what was officially "family time." Hank agreed to let me meet Oz and his kids at the park. Tallulah was going to a friend's house, but she asked me, "Why are you spending time with Oz again?" I explained that he was a "special friend of mine who I was reconnecting with." Tallulah had been watching me closely since I'd started dating Oz; I sensed she felt a shift in me. But I felt good about what I was doing. I had grown up with a depressed mother who I was frequently caretaking. I was making myself happy without burdening my kids—I could keep it all under control.

This was our first playdate with the kids. Amy and Merlin were so young, at three and five, that they just thought of it as a good time. And Liam and Merlin were friends from school, so it was normal for them to play together. Oz had boundless energy playing with our kids. I loved his comfortable exuberance. I had bought small water pistols for Merlin and Liam; Amy got a smaller gun, and Oz got the smallest. I had purchased for myself a double-barrel half-gallon Uzi. I explained apologetically to Oz that they ran out of the big guns and that's why I bought him a smaller one.

"Oh really? It seems very suspicious that they had only one Uzi water gun." Oz stood holding his tiny pistol.

"It is odd," I replied with sympathy.

Then Oz sprayed me with his gun and we ran through the park squirting each other. Oz grabbed my Uzi and doused me. But I insisted he stop—frizzy hair was unfair combat.

We stopped to eat sandwiches on the picnic bench. Then Liam and Merlin ran off to the swings. I was happy our kids were having so much fun together. I blew bubbles for Amy, who chased them in the air till they landed gently on the grass. Oz took the wand, dipped it in the soapy water, and then blew a huge bubble for Amy, who shrieked in glee. Then Oz casually commented that he had been scouting single-parent meet-ups and that they felt oddly like dating sites.

Whoa, Tonto. I felt a cold breeze of fear as my heart constricted.

"You are so lucky you have Hank," Oz continued. "I feel so worried for Susan. The dating scene is so abysmal for us."

My brain came to a full stop. *Us? What do you mean, "us"?* I consciously urged myself to breathe deeper. Merlin called for Oz to throw him the football. Oz bent over to pick it up, flashing his hot pink silk thong as he leaned down. Oz's pants hung low revealing his taut abs. I suddenly imagined single women at a meet-up with the same view.

"Hey! It's called a B-E-L-T! I am ordering you one online."

I reached for my cell phone and Googled men's belts. Oz threw the football to the boys. It soared through the air spinning, then landed a good fifty feet out. Liam and Merlin ran to it.

I am not ready to share you. Fuck all the poly rules. I felt flustered. What was happening to the Queen of Compersion? I was *jealous.*

On our next date, Oz described needing to feel "in control." He couldn't control when he saw me or his kids.

"I just spent two years trying to negotiate the right to love whomever I want—mainly you. But I need to feel that I can have another lover if I choose to."

We had been dating a little over a month—now he wanted to sleep around. When we first got together we agreed to be exclusive to each other for six months. I had never dwelled on the idea or even the possibility that Oz would even want to see other women when the six months were up. It seemed like a miniscule, distant, possible reality. But now listening to Oz talk about dating other women inflicted a deep vat of dread in my belly. For the past month I was ecstatic to be having sex with Oz. I was in a process of sexual self-discovery. I was getting a blend of what I wanted most—sex and love together. But Oz wanting to date made me feel emotionally unsafe.

That night I called Reenie.

She chuckled, "Isn't that what poly is—he gets to date?"

Reenie sounded a bit satisfied that I had run amok.

"True," I said, "But we agreed on a six-month period to build a foundation."

"Sounds like that's not his timing."

Her tone unnerved me a bit. It seemed like even my friends wanted me to pick a set of rules and follow them.

Over the next two weeks, Oz became increasingly forlorn when he was by himself. I would get agonizing texts:

I need someone of my own. You have Hank. I want someone too.

Oz was shaken by Hank's retracting overnights. But I felt I couldn't push Hank to reconsider right now; he was at his limit.

I asked Oz to wait until we were on stronger footing. I reminded him of our original agreement, but he missed family life and didn't seem to tolerate being alone. I wanted more time to build trust with Oz. After that I could imagine being more adventurous in terms of having an open relationship. But I needed a stronger bond before contemplating that. Also, given my history of struggling to integrate passion and love, Oz's sexuality was a bit frightening to me. Oz was a wild card. I had asked for love and sexuality—now, having both in one man, I found myself almost in a crisis. I needed more time to acclimate to our highly sexual connection.

Finally, Oz represented what I did not want to happen to me—he had lost his mate. I was afraid of doing the same and destabilizing my life. Although I trusted myself to handle whatever happened, losing people reminded me of the chaos of my childhood. Going slow was the path of self-preservation for me. The fact that Oz would not slow down set off alarm bells.

On our next date at his apartment, things got worse. On my quest for emotional safety, I asked Oz every minute detail about his relations with women and ex-girlfriends. I found it endearing that he'd slept with only five women, but a few minutes into the conversation this number doubled to ten. After further questioning, one could arguably add another dozen women. Apparently there were ten women who waved the go flag, and then about ten more that Oz had "sort of slept with." This included one woman who allowed Oz to rub the tip of his penis an inch into her labia, moving up and down for nearly thirty minutes!

"Really?" I asked incredulous. It sounded both fantastic and weird. "After five minutes she didn't ask you to take it on home? What amazing foreplay."

"She said we couldn't have sex."

"Hello! Last I checked rubbing the tip of your penis in a woman's vagina qualifies as sex."

Then Oz revealed more sexual skeletons. Apparently Oz had a little hobby of visiting strip clubs. My brain screeched to a halt. *Where was the sweet, reserved librarian?* I gulped.

"I've only visited—maybe fifteen clubs."

I felt slightly light-headed, my chest tightening. Oz noticed the change that had come over me. He misinterpreted it.

"You're such a prude. So I occasionally go to a strip club."

"That's not it," I murmured.

I was terrified—*Oz visited strip clubs!*—he was a sexist brute. He was a bad boy, he was a good boy, he was a librarian, he was a man-ho. *Could I tolerate both? Was it safe to tolerate both?*

"Can we talk about what you are thinking and feeling?"

"You want my feminist lecture?"

"You fascinate me. You're my muse. I learn a lot when we talk about these things."

We kept talking. But all of it—the strip clubs, the lovers multiplying from five to twenty, his urgency to date other women—unnerved me. Oz called me his "breakthrough person" who ushered him into a world in which he was growing emotionally. He was both afraid and intrigued to date again. He wanted me to be his support system. But I could easily see getting used up if I had to coddle Oz through dating other women. The whole notion made me shudder. After several more conversations, I pointed out the disparity in our situation.

"You are my only lover. Hank and I aren't having sex. I am monogamous to you."

"Yes, but you live with him. I have limited access to you, whereas you have Hank and your kids all the time."

When Oz expressed fear about how alone he felt in the world, I felt annoyed. He had wealth that provided plenty of resources and time to rebuild his life. What could possibly be his problem? I had reinvented myself many times alone—with no money, no safety net, no family. I didn't have much empathy for Oz. Why couldn't he wait?

But Oz was anxiety ridden and wearing down, so I told him to make me a voice memo of exactly what he needed. The next week I was going to Passover back east with Hank and my kids. We agreed I'd listen to it on my trip.

I approached the trip to Boston in the way that I imagined a closeted homosexual in the 1950s approaching a family visit—clinging to the closet and dreading coming out. Although I still held fast to the innovative way we were setting up our relationship, the thought of outing myself to Hank's family sent a cold chill up my vertebrae. Hank and I agreed to keep it on the down low. He was afraid too. He told me his father would more likely understand his robbing a bank than opening his marriage. But I was sure that when the truth came out I'd get panned more than Hank. Although we shared much love, I feared that everyone would likely suspect me as the initiator. I'd always had an unwilling transparency.

When I was pregnant with each of my kids, the hormones affected me like a feline overdosed on catnip. This was in the days of dial-up Internet connections. When I tried to get relief with some porn, I'd wait agonizing minutes for images of cock that were then almost instantly snatched away. This drove me to rent videos at a local sex shop. The young women at the front desk never got tired of teasing me as I shamefully plunked down my pile of videos. "Girl! This is how you got knocked up in the first place!" Humor hath no better target like a horny pregnant woman. I stood alone—a chubby libidinous anomaly. The men in the store would stare at me as if they'd spotted a Martian. It was uncomfortable to say the least. I would beg Hank to return my videos for me. Sometimes we'd go in together, me shaking my head, playing the victimized pregnant wife, standing by her man with his nasty porn addiction.

"He said he'd buy me a burger after we returned the videos," my sad little eyes would say to the customers milling about.

But there were no sad little eyes for me from Hank's family. They, like everyone else, just seemed to know what a horny gal I was. I was not ready to be potentially burned at the stake. In my lifetime they were my first taste of a loving, stable family, and over the years I had leaped many hurdles to gain their acceptance. Just last year, at a wedding with Hank's family, we had missed the exodus of the hired taxi. So Hank's Uncle Ezra gave us a ride. There weren't enough seat belts for the kids and Hank and me. We stood around the car troubleshooting. I was adamant that the kids have both lap and sash belts. Uncle Ezra, who was generally impatient, stood running scenarios with me. I knew how annoyed he was. After ten minutes I decided that I'd be the one to fly through the windshield and skid on the road if there was a collision. I lay down in the back of the station wagon (the only way I could fit) while we drove the two miles to the hotel.

The next day, sipping champagne under the ceremonial tent, Uncle Ezra piped up out of nowhere, "You're a great mom!" I received this compliment like manna from God.

My own parents had never met my children and were now dead. I had no desire to lose my adoptive parents by revealing that we'd opened our marriage.

We stepped off the plane in the late afternoon. When we arrived at Hank's cousin's house, it was packed with relatives. We had the top attic floor all to ourselves. That evening we drank wine, played scrabble, and ate roasted chicken.

The next morning, while everyone was downstairs making breakfast, I sat down to listen to Oz's voice memo. I did some deep breathing, sending a cord deep into the earth. I pressed play. When I heard Oz's voice, my heart melted, then lurched. He started out quietly, saying that his primary wish was "to grow our relationship." I took a deep breath.

Then he began his list of desires. He wanted to be able to have sex with any of the women he had previously had sex with. *Great*—by Oz's definition of "sex" this could be anywhere from ten to fifty women. He listed an old girlfriend. I took a deep breath. He wanted to seek out two women who "got away" years ago and romance them. I felt my heart sink. He mentioned two women friends he was sexually attracted to and wanted to spend more time with. He also said he was interested in going to some sex parties, and would I like to come along?

Fantastic. This was shaping up to be a really horrific cocktail. There was more. He wanted to experience a one-night stand, picking up a woman he didn't know to have sex with her. His list of requests felt like a verbal bat repeatedly beating me. He went on, but I was getting that spacey feeling again—as if my head were floating away. The voice memo in its entirety was about six minutes long, but by the end of it I sat slumped in the Barcalounger I'd claimed as my meditation chair. I was bonked on cortisol like one of those marathon runners after a really long uphill climb. The room suddenly felt stuffy. I had to get out and move. I walked on wobbly legs down the steep attic steps.

"Anyone want to go for a run?!" I announced.

Hank looked up from his scrambled eggs and matzo, his eyes frozen on me for a second. *Did I sound shrill?* I clutched my cell phone.

"All righty! I am off!"

I started sprinting toward the bike path and dialing at the same time. *Please be home, please be home.* Reenie picked up as I ran down the gravel incline toward the wide paved trail.

"Hey!" she said.

"He wants to fuck everyone!"

"What?" I was usually the stable good listener. But lately when I called my friends they snapped into an alert, attentive state.

"I thought he was this sweet, shy librarian. But he wants to fuck every woman he's ever met—and more!"

"Slow down, take some breaths."

"I know I am supposed to use these feelings to evolve myself. That's the poly creed on jealousy. It all sounded so good on paper."

While Reenie listened quietly, I could hear myself. I sounded like I was on speed. I started to run again.

"Reenie, I feel so loved and the sex is amazing—but if he needs to date other women—"

My voice trailed off. I felt embarrassed that I didn't want Oz to date. I had sold everyone on poly, and now I was doing an about-face. I ran by a father pushing his twins in a stroller; he cautiously glanced at me. I had become one of those people you took sneak peeks at, the village wild woman.

"That's great that the sex is so good. But after menopause you may not feel the same way about Oz. It's important to maintain what you have in your marriage."

I was now walking at a steady clip. Maybe she was right. But people were always trying to convince me that dick was not all that important—and maybe it wasn't to them. But I had a hard time believing there'd come a day when I just didn't care. We talked until I was calmer. Then I went back to the house and started washing the breakfast dishes for the family. Hank came in to hang out with me.

"Oh, by the way, Oz's mother wants to have lunch with me. She's going to pick me up in a few hours."

"What?" Hank had that slow, simmering look.

I stammered, "Oz's parents live nearby and his mother wants to have lunch," my voice trailed off.

"You didn't ask me."

I felt a vise of anxiety in my chest—another poly nightmare.

"I guess I forgot to ask. I didn't think it would be such a big deal." We went back and forth.

"Should I cancel?" I asked.

"You made plans and never cleared them."

"That was stupid. I wasn't thinking."

Hank didn't say much more.

Oz's mother, Monica, came an hour later and met Hank, Tallulah, and Merlin at the door. Hank's eyes were flashing, a bead of sweat was on his brow. I was a first-class poly failure. *Get permission weeks before—years before!*

We headed off in her SUV. I was barely able to concentrate on the conversation because of my internal drone, a chorus yelling at me of my poly failings. After a short ride, we arrived at her home. We parked in front of a four-story Victorian with a widow's walk. Inside there were tapestries and original art all done by Monica. The kitchen cabinet doors had been replaced by vibrantly colored Indian screens.

We ate a beet salad and a tomato-based clam chowder, from yellow china that Monica said was a wedding gift forty years prior. As we spooned our chowder, we exchanged observations about Oz. I shared how, when I'd first met him, he loathed the idea of being kind to himself or meditating or any kind of internal exploration. Monica told me that Oz's fathers and grandfather's families seemed to be dominated by intellectual giants, very successful geeks.

"Our family lineage values the intellect above all else," said Monica.

But she explained that in the past decade she'd been exploring spirituality, emotions, and intuition. After lunch she showed me the carriage house that she'd renovated into her art studio. Many more of her tapestries hung on the walls. I loved all her art: the mythological imagery, fully pregnant women, and amazons doing archery. I was very struck by our similarities. When she dropped me back at the house we hugged and promised to meet again soon.

She said, "There's a lot that you clearly have to teach Oz and the world as well."

I stepped out of the car and immediately went in search of Hank, who I found in the backyard smoking.

"Why are you smoking again?"

"Oh, gee, let me think. My life is feeling a bit stressful lately. Could that be it?"

"If you don't stop, I am going to tell your family you're smoking."

"If you tell them I'm smoking, I'm gonna tell them *why* I'm smoking."

We both laughed, which momentarily eased the tension. But a knot was forming in my stomach. From experience with Hank, I knew still waters could mean angry sharks were lurking. Hank was conflict avoidant, but I was anxious over what could possibly be coming. If Hank continued to be unhappy, I didn't know what I'd do.

The next morning I woke up early and climbed into the meditation Barcalounger. I asked for guidance, then sat breathing. A new thought came to me. *I don't have to date Oz while he sees other women.* I had this image of me getting off the Oz train, waving to Oz, and wishing him luck as he continued on his journey. I felt instant relief in my body.

Oz seemed to be on a different poly journey—and I wasn't sure our needs were currently compatible. I wanted the depth of our new connection to be the priority. I had met men in the poly world that seemed high on the idea of new ass whenever they wanted it. If this was what Oz needed, I had to let him go, at least for now. I was not interested in sexual experiences that were like addictive substances. I could possibly see stretching my boundaries by our going to sex parties together—but only after building a foundation in which I felt safe. I would not stand in Oz's way. He could explore polyamory his way. Just without me. We could check in after a time-out. I needed energy to be present for my kids and my life and not be stressing about who Oz was fucking. I gave thanks for the epiphany.

We arrived home late at night. Hank had stopped talking to me. He put up a good front around his family, but when we boarded the plane he was silent. When Hank was hurt, I felt like I was trapped in a dark forest during a storm. He was a man of few words, but he did manage to communicate to me "I feel betrayed" and that we might need a divorce, something he had never mentioned before. Then he barely spoke to me. Even though I knew I could handle being alone, it was my worst-case scenario. *What if I lose Hank?* We had carried each other through both crisis and triumph for the past twenty-five years—I couldn't even imagine a life without him in it; the family we'd created together was my constancy.

The next day I limped over to him while he quietly shaved in the bathroom.

"I feel like I am losing you," I shared.

It was a stark overcast morning. Hank was at his most self-contained as he watched his reflection in the mirror.

"I don't want to lose you or our family or your parents or every-one in Boston." I was sobbing now, overcome by my own vulnerability.

My life with Hank flashed before my eyes. *Why should we throw away a relationship when most of it worked?* That was a script for someone else's life. I had friends whose spouses had been piggy and mean, even violent. When they finally woke up they couldn't get divorced fast enough. But that wasn't my life. If there was any hard-earned wisdom here it was simply not to idealize anyone, and to know that all things change, including what you may need from a spouse.

I wanted to retain all the good things: our love, our friendship, our financial enterprises, our co-parenting. It was the civilized and evolved thing to do. It was my vision, and I was wedded to it like a devoted bride, starry eyed and willing to go to any lengths to make it happen.

Things were touch and go for the rest of the week. On day five, I consulted one of my divination tools, the I Ching. Literally meaning "the book of change," it is one of the oldest books ever written. When I asked about my relationship with Hank, I got the hexagram "Creative Power," saying that worthwhile goals will result in "sublime success." My eyes welled up with tears as I descended the stairs to find Hank drinking his morning cup of coffee. I read from the book.

Hank smiled. He could see how moved I was.

"You put a lot of weight in the I Ching," he said.

"I put a lot of weight in us," I replied.

Something transpired after that. Very slowly we tiptoed out of that dark place where one false move meant we'd lose each other. It's hard to say even now what made it better. But Hank could feel that his presence held a huge significance for me, even though I still loved Oz. I got something different and vital from Hank. Somehow going to the precipice and backing up, Hank allowed me more space to have Oz.

That weekend Hank okayed an overnight. I told Hank all the turmoil I was having with Oz possibly dating other women. He was empathetic and even protective of me. It was striking to have these conversations with my husband about my new love, but I was gratified that Hank was rooting for me too. Oz and I decided to go to Tomales Bay. I told Tallulah I was going on a retreat with Aurora, who had become my beard when I was with Oz. Merlin was fine with the overnight, but Tallulah looked at me with squinty eyes of suspicion.

On the way out of town, Oz and I stopped at a sex shop on Polk Street. Oz asked me if I'd feel exploited if he bought me a pair of thigh-high lace-up boots. I reassured him there was nothing I liked better than industrial-strength slut gear. We bought the boots and two negligees. Then we were off across the Golden Gate Bridge and up the coast. We checked into our hotel. It was pouring rain and we got drenched running to our room. Inside we tore off each other's clothes and fell into bed, making love urgently, then more slowly the second time, after I'd modeled the boots for him. We were wrapped tightly around each other under the sheets.

"Hey," I said, pulling away. "We need to talk."

"Okay." Oz stuffed some pillows under his head.

"I want to discuss your voice memo."

When I came home from back east, I was deluged with the crisis with Hank. And for the next several days after the trip that's all I spoke about to Oz. All I had said in response to his long voice mail was that we could "work something out" and let's "talk about it this weekend." Now was the moment to sort things out.

"There's something you should know about me. I really evaluate situations. I've had so much chaos as a kid, I developed a side to me that is very self-preserving—"

"Grace, I am so anxious right now. What's going on?"

"It's just—if you want to see other women, I'd need a time-out from us."

Oz leaned back against the pillows and smiled at me. "The most important thing to me is to be connected to you."

"But it sounds like you want to date other women. You could make an OkCupid page, date poly women, and see where you land. We could meet back up in three months."

"I'd miss you too much. I've been through too much to have you."

"Oh, baby."

I nestled into his chest. I took a deep inhale of his body— somewhere between soap and musky pine needles. We held each other quietly, but I wasn't sure this had been so easily resolved.

The next day we packed up Oz's silver Fiat. I wanted to make love one more time in the room, but Oz wanted to go home and make love at his place. We headed up Highway 101 through a torrential downpour. I drove because Oz's SI joint was acting up. We chatted, meandering through conversation with no particular agenda. We reviewed the past week, my dilemma with Hank, my panic that I would be divorced and in the same place Oz was. Oz casually launched into a free-association monologue describing his feelings.

"Yes, I was scared too, hearing how hard things were between you and Hank. 'Oh great!' I thought. 'If Hank leaves Grace then I'll have to be monogamous with her.'"

Huh? My whole being sat up.

"Then I thought, 'Oh, God, that would be worse than being monogamous with Susan.' I mean, you're an emotional sports car—Susan is more a minivan. At least with a minivan I'm investing in a model that has longevity to bank on. When I took last year off to look for a better job, our bank account was still going up and up and up."

I sat mute. I had noted this quality in Oz, a kind of open-mouth-stick-in-foot syndrome. Oz occasionally made miscalculations as to the effect of his words. He had what the Irish would call "a touch of the Asperger's." I was speechless and suddenly numb. A voice pierced my brain like a loud speaker at some raucous public event: *Collect yourself, make small talk. Get back to your people and describe exactly in precise detail what you just heard. Then await further instructions.*

I made small talk. Then I had a feeling wash over me that I can only describe in one verb: *Escape!* I had promised Tallulah that I would take her to a movie when I returned from my overnight. A homesick feeling came over me. I longed to be with Tallulah, Hank, and Merlin. Oz sat next to me describing some intricate parallel world of his experience.

"Hey," I said casually. "Would you mind if I went home early instead of going back to your place?"

"Sure, we can do that," Oz's brow slightly furrowed.

A few moments later, in a distinctly quieter car, Oz asked, "Could we spend a little time at my place? When do you need to be home?"

What to do? What to say? My heart and soul felt a million miles away. My body wanted to follow. I have always been embarrassed by money—humiliated by it. As a child I felt like I was a drain on my mother's finances merely by existing. I was proud of my work as a Pilates instructor, and I thought I was doing fine financially, but I wasn't making Oz bucks. Hearing that I was being measured by this yardstick and found lacking was devastating. If that wasn't enough, there was his dismal reaction to possibly having me available full-time. It made me want to press the intercom to the mother ship and wail, "Scotty! Beam me up!"

What was I doing to my life? Was polyamory an absolutely crazy lifestyle? I was clearly creating havoc in my marriage, and for what? Oz didn't seem to value "us." I drove on in silence.

Oz asked again, "Can we spend more time together?"

Against all better judgment I answered honestly.

"You know, I think I am having a response to what you said about being monogamous with me, that you would 'dread' that."

We went back and forth.

Then I voiced my concerns again, "I'm glad you were honest, so at the very least I can protect myself."

Oz groaned, then fearfully looked out the window, then back at me. His eyes darted around the car; then he actually started crying. *Oh no, we're really in it now. Process station! Your train will be delayed for at least an hour, realistically more like two. Another fucking poly processing nightmare! Wasn't this supposed to be my vacation?*

When we got back to Oz's penthouse (but still at Process Station) Oz reassured me that my poverty status was not a problem for him. In fact, Oz said he was contemplating changing his will to include me.

He said, "This last week you've been putting down poly every time I talked to you. But if you put down poly, you are putting down our relationship."

"I am sorry. I'm not putting you down. I'm struggling with poly…"

I needed a break to think. I could see Oz was struggling too.

I went home to Hank.

"Check this out," I announced to Hank. Then I gave him a blow-by-blow description of my ride home with Oz.

"Poly sucks," I concluded.

"What did you expect it to be? Like one of those *Star Trek* episodes where they land on a Utopian planet and all the fruit is ripe and succulent and plentiful?"

"Yes! That's exactly what I expected it to be!"

"Don't you remember there was always a scary monster that needed to be fed?"

"Poly creates as many problems as it solves."

The poly ride was now feeling like a lousy dating situation. Was I being ungrateful? Poly had allowed me to experience sexual ecstasy and love with Oz—while keeping Hank. If the ride stopped here I'd get off the train with so many treasured memories. But everything felt unmoored. Poly felt like a disappointment—at least that day. It was like Hank said, *There was always someone a little pissed off at you.* In my exuberance to reconfigure my life, it hadn't occurred to me how complex it would be to make so many people happy. It didn't occur to me that my actions might hurt or upset other people who I'd have to eventually nurse back to normalcy, including myself. That night I fell into a deep sleep, relieved to be at least momentarily in another world.

Chapter 13

When I told Oz that if he wanted to go on an all-out man-ho excursion I would have to disembark from the train, the urgency of his needs shifted. Things slowed down; we edged around how to move forward. One night after making love, Oz tried to sell me again.

"I would date someone completely different from you—ethnically, emotionally."

But I wanted to be more primary to Oz. I wanted Oz to invest in me first. I wanted him to wait to add in other people. I realized that one of the things that had enabled me to do poly with Hank was all the years of trust and foundation that we'd built. I wanted a partner who would close our relationship if need be, to preserve it. But if Oz felt our relationship wasn't worth investing in, then I wanted him to go off and explore on his own. I rolled on my side and wrapped the blankets around me. I knew this was going to end badly.

"Please don't go away." Oz pulled me back into his chest. "I don't want to do anything that will make you turn away from me."

The next morning, when Hank and I were drinking our coffee, a dozen roses arrived by courier.

"Did you and Oz have a fight?"

I opened the card. It read:

You are my perfect woman... Oz

"I don't think we had a fight."

Hank watched me put the long-stemmed roses into a vase.

"Oh, you two had a fight all right."

As I trimmed the roses, I described my dilemma. I wasn't ready for Oz to date other women, but as a solution I might be willing to go to sex parties with Oz, be a swinger couple.

"Could you sign off on that?"

Hank drank his coffee quietly, then said, "Didn't you write on your OkCupid profile that you didn't want to date men who go to sex parties? Now you want to go to one with Oz? What's going on?"

What had changed was that I was finally getting love and sex from one source. My connection to Oz felt significant; the only other time I'd been this deeply in love was with Hank. I didn't want Oz to dilute our growing connection with a few more girlfriends; and I knew from experience with Valerie and Hank's relationship that Oz's theoretical girlfriend would have her own set of demands and needs. A large part of me wanted to keep the focus on growing "us." But I was possibly open to "play parties," which would be about sexual exploration, not long-term ties. Some poly friends had invited me to their play party—which was not quite an orgy, but would be held in a place with separate rooms where people could talk privately, make out, or engage in sexual activities.

My life felt too complicated to add more people into my world. I could foresee a season in the future in which I might be more open, but right now I'd rather spend the time with my kids and my friends. Frankly, the thought of adding even one more person—one more psyche, one more set of needs, one more complication—made me want to lock myself in a closet with a pitcher of martinis.

But I was attempting to stretch my comfort zone to keep Oz. In the swinger lifestyle, you could play at a party and never see the person again. But there was the sure reality that after the sex party, I'd claw Oz's face off. *You stared at her breasts too long!* I reasoned that with a few hours of emotional processing and some Bactine we'd make it through the clawing part of the evening. But Hank nailed it. Was that really the best choice here?

However, that week, when I was pondering how to handle Oz, things exploded at home. Tallulah had become increasingly suspicious. We had been successfully keeping it all under wraps. But when I started seeing Oz, it tipped the applecart. Suddenly all my cover stories seemed flimsy. I was "going out with friends," I had to "teach an evening class." As I prepared for a date, I'd turn to see Tallulah watching me put on my mascara at my vanity. She was the canary in the coal mine, whiffing change in the air.

We thought we were pulling off the facade for now. When they were older we'd explain more. But at ten years old, Tallulah was an old soul, with a searing intelligence and a formidable presence. Her facile brain was quick to assess a situation. She began to ask more questions about our friendships.

During breakfast Tallulah drilled us further about our "special friends." We explained that sometimes in a marriage you made friends of the opposite sex and that this "added to your life." We thought we were pretty damn smart and this would be a satisfying answer.

But Tallulah asked us directly, "Are you having sex?"

I was taken aback. But I piped up gamely, "We may sometimes kiss each other."

Tallulah burst into tears. I met Hank's gaze across the platter of bagels. What I saw there mirrored my own feelings. *We are over our heads. Swim for shore!* Panicked, we told Tallulah we wouldn't kiss our "special friends" any more.

That night Hank and I holed up in the sunroom. We were now united in this new onslaught. We looked at each other, then started to giggle because, quite frankly, it felt like a bad acid trip.

"Let me off the spaceship," Hank said.

"What should we do? Who can we call?" I was truly baffled.

What I knew about Tallulah was that she asked questions like a twenty-six-year-old but could only handle answers appropriate for a ten-year-old. We kept giving her our ten-year-old answers, but over the next few weeks Tallulah began to watch us even more closely. She sensed that we were not giving her the straight scoop.

A week later things went from bad to worse. Feeling Tallulah's eyes upon me, I decided to change the password on my cell phone…

just in case. But when I left the room one afternoon, she grabbed it off the table where I had set it down after using it. The lock system hadn't activated. She started reading my texts. I was doing dishes in the kitchen when she started wailing. I ran into the room. She had my cell phone open to an amorous text from Oz. *Good Goddess the jig was up!* I called Hank and left him a voice mail. Tallulah collapsed on the couch sobbing. My precocious child had read too much.

"Are you having sex with Oz?" she cried.

I had to tell the truth.

"Yes," I answered.

I tried to comfort her. But she was having none of it. The girl was seriously scared. My heart felt like a lead weight. *What am I doing? Am I destroying my family?* I canceled all my clients and took her walking in the hills. I was struck by how I had not seen this coming. I spent my whole childhood helping my mother. She had been depressed and unstable after her second divorce. I never saw her in a happy relationship. This was my burden as a child; I wanted my mother to be happy. I thought I was gifting Tallulah with a happy mother, being proactive about getting my needs met.

Hank arrived home by the end of our walk. I basically kept asking Tallulah what she needed. She said for "everything to be the same." My heart sank. We gave Hank a report, then Tallulah started crying again.

"At least Daddy and Valerie don't have sex," she commanded.

My gaze met Hank's over Tallulah's head.

My eyes said, *Dude, don't you dare sell me out.*

Hank gently told Tallulah that he and Valerie were more than special friends. Poor Tallulah cried fresh tears. It seemed like her whole world was collapsing. I texted Oz an SOS; he called immediately. I gave him an update on the misery at hand.

He thought a moment, then said, "All we can do is love our kids the best we can."

Good Lilith, platitudes. What the hell am I going to do?

Then Oz suggested calling the famous author who'd written *the book* on poly. She had a counseling practice in San Francisco. I did an Internet search for her phone number, then booked an appointment for the next evening.

We arrived at our session with great expectation. Fantastic! Someone was going to tell us what to do. Our counselor, a friendly woman in her sixties, sat us down. We laid out our story about Tallulah's response to our "special friends." We explained that Merlin was five years old and for him Oz and Valerie were just fun new playmates.

We asked our expert how to help our kids adjust. She had raised her child in a polyamorous family. Her daughter, a physician in New York City, was now in her thirties. Clearly, she hadn't screwed up her kid. But soon it became obvious that our expert's situation as a parent was vastly different from ours. She was part of a commune in the early '70s. Polyamory and communal living was all her daughter ever knew. Our counselor told us stories of dozens of poly parents in the commune. She had lived in a Utopian fuckfest. But how were we supposed to help Tallulah? She suggested we "be confident" and not doubt "our decisions and value system." She encouraged us to reassure Tallulah and help her through the transitions as we would in any other difficult transition. But this was different than any other transition I'd experienced as a parent. Only slightly bolstered, we went to pick up Merlin and Tallulah from Valerie's loft, where she had volunteered to watch them.

Tallulah got into the car and put on her seat belt.

"How did it go?" she asked us.

Hank started out. "It went very well, honey. We learned a lot."

"Oh, yes? Like what?" asked Tallulah.

We told Tallulah how much we loved her. She and Merlin—who sat gazing out the window, oblivious—were our number-one priority. We reassured her that we were devoted to her and that was not going to change. Then we went on to describe our poly philosophy, which was turning out to be the integration of Oz and Valerie into our family. Our special friends were chosen family and wonderful additions to our life. We had a shortage of family; Valerie and Oz would allow us to spend more quality time together.

"That doesn't make sense. How can going off on dates two nights a week increase our family time together?"

Tallulah went on rapid fire, a mini Johnnie Cochran poking holes in our vision. She wanted to know what was happening with me and Hank. She was also concerned that we wouldn't have time for her.

She concluded, "I hate poly. I don't think you should be doing it."

We were both dumbstruck.

After a pause, Hank said, with a buttressed attempt at a confident delivery, "I'm glad we talked about this. We'll talk more another time."

We glanced at each other, two startled colts, spooked by a wildcat. I was having my doubts about how to do poly with Oz. In fact, I was beginning to think of polyamory and monogamy as points on a spectrum. I was using the term "poly" when what I really meant was "innovation in relationship"—having many choices of how to set up a relationship. For me, poly was about building a deep emotional connection in which you could create current agreements that reflected everyone's needs. But I was still sorting this all out, and it was disconcerting—to say the least—to have my ten-year-old daughter interrogating me, listing the very fears that I was still grappling with. Now that Tallulah was afraid and presenting her case, I was wondering again if poly—or this process of innovation in my relationships—was worth it.

I called Oz after I'd put the kids to bed. I told him it was a complete bust. He said he'd found a class in the city—an evening workshop discussing how to create poly families. I got off the phone and told Hank about it. He was eager to hear what they would teach us.

A few evenings later, on our date night, Oz and I attended the workshop on poly families. We introduced ourselves as novices to poly who were trying to make it work for us and our kids. We went around the circle, each person introducing him- or herself. Out of the seven couples, we were the only ones with kids! Over the next hour, the group leader kept saying things like, "I read about this poly family in Arizona…"

At one point a young man sitting next to Oz piped up, "Can we hear how it is working for both of you, since you're the only ones with children?"

Out of everyone, we were the closest to "experts." When they passed around the donation basket, Oz whispered in my ear, "I am so not paying for this workshop." We left early.

The poly books talked about your relationships with all your partners. But who knew how to help with the kids? I worried about my connection with Tallulah. We were so close, but this was a wedge between us. I absolutely couldn't lose the bond with my daughter.

Luckily one of my closest pals happened to be a child psychologist. Freya became a huge resource both in terms of child development and poly philosophy. Freya lived with her ex-husband, who was one of her best friends. Her lesbian partners understood her desire to stay connected with a former lover and create chosen family. Freya agreed with the poly expert, although she acknowledged that her advice had sounded trite. Freya suggested I explain our "vision" and reassure Tallulah that it would be okay. I had to sit with myself, getting clear on how to describe my vision to Tallulah. Basically it came down to Tallulah and Merlin (and Oz's children) thriving while we integrated our new partners into our lives—creating more family.

When I discussed my vision with Freya, she understood the desire for chosen family but explained that, at ten years old, Tallulah was very focused on fitting in with her peers. Our family choices were most likely making her feel different. Freya also suggested I find out what Tallulah was most afraid of so that we could actively help alleviate her fears.

During this time, Freya became one of the few people who really understood how I was feeling. After I had come back from the Passover disaster vacation, I had confessed to her that I felt like a poly fraud. I felt sorry for the false advertising with Oz: *When you leave your marriage, you can have me and any other woman you want!* Although I had not quite said that to Oz, I was sure he thought that would happen. I confided to Freya that I felt I couldn't do the sexual poly thing, at least not to the extent that Oz seemed to want to do it.

Freya told me she felt the same way. In the world of multiple sexual partners, an emotionally sensitive soul could feel like she was going through a relationship meat grinder. But there were parts of the poly doctrine that still resonated with me. I loved the whole concept of honesty within relationships, which included taking responsibility for your feelings and happiness. The sex-positive aspect of the poly world was very appealing; normalizing attractions to other people felt like a huge relief. I also liked the idea of staying current about needs and making agreements that worked for both parties. I loved the authenticity of integrating all parts of your being on a relationship journey.

Freya and I coined the term "emotional poly" for what we were doing: a state wherein you stay close and loving with former sexual partners. That was what she had done with her former husband, who was now family to her. This was very inspiring to me. But she warned me that although her lesbian lovers thought it was a grand setup, the heterosexual women who dated her former husband were very ambivalent about Freya. They felt threatened by Freya's intimate emotional connection with her former husband.

I decided to take Tallulah to a session with my longtime therapist, Judy. I wanted a calm space to talk with Tallulah. Tallulah's anger at me was intimidating. Since reading my text from Oz she had stopped talking to me when I got ready for my dates and would not kiss me good-bye, which unnerved me considerably. As we drove to Judy's office she barked from the backseat of the car, "She better be a good therapist—not like that woman in San Francisco."

I needed a supportive witness. I wanted to see how Judy would handle Tallulah's hostility. But when we arrived, Tallulah did her charming-kitten act, talking in soft tones, complimenting Judy's office decor.

"Is that statue an African fertility symbol?" she asked quietly as she settled into the couch.

Damn it. No one ever saw what I was dealing with.

Judy was impressed with Tallulah's articulate maturity. During the session Tallulah explained, "I like Oz. I just don't like what Mom is doing with Oz."

We explored some of Tallulah's fears that Daddy and Mommy would get a divorce and that the changes would hurt us as a family. At the end of the session, Judy encouraged me to spend more quality time with Tallulah, to reassure her of our bond.

In the next few weeks I ramped up our "special time" together with shopping trips, walks, snuggling on Sunday afternoons, and watching movies. But the more attention I gave Tallulah, the more she demanded. She talked down to me like I was an imbecilic teenager screwing up my life. I was trying to pull off my vision of transforming my life, and Tallulah was all over my ass. In hindsight I can say that being blessed with a highly emotionally intelligent kid keeps a mother on her toes. Tallulah could assess a situation and intuit what was about to happen before I could even foresee it.

There was also another dynamic at play. Tallulah was picking up on the areas I was insecure about and hammering away at them. If I had figured this out at the time, I might have created a private space to ponder my next move without Tallulah interrogating me. From where I sit now, I am proud of what I've modeled for Tallulah: resourcefulness, adhering to your own vision, and being a woman (and mother) willing to put yourself high on the priority list of people who mattered. But at the time I was mightily intimidated by her interrogations.

And because some of Tallulah's fears were my fears, I was daunted by them. She needed stability and I did too. Things with Oz had gotten too drama filled, and somewhere along the way my grand plan of getting laid and having my intact family was unraveling.

A month after Tallulah got into my cell phone, we were still trying to stabilize the situation. One Saturday Oz and I took our kids to Jumpy Town, a large gymnasium filled with inflatable bouncy houses. Tallulah decided she was too old for this and so she spent the afternoon with a friend.

Oz and I were in the biggest fun house, leaping up and down. Merlin and Liam ran off to do the obstacle course with Amy.

Oz said, "I have something to tell you."

I spiked with a moment of terror. *Is he about to tell me he's slept with another woman?* He told me that he had met a woman while getting a slice of pizza. They'd chatted it up. She told him about her bipolar diagnosis and Oz told her that he was poly. It was a spontaneous confessional. Oz described me by saying he was "in love" with me. She told him he was "really cute" and that if he'd ever consider being monogamous to give her a call.

We were surrounded by a dozen kids exuberantly leaping and hollering. I could barely hear myself think. I felt exhausted by more drama. Even though he didn't stick it to anyone else, the fact that he'd flirted with and desired another woman made me feel almost as lousy.

I tried to remain neutral and discern Oz's needs.

"Timing is a really important part of communication," I began. "What was your intention in telling me this?"

Yet, as I questioned him I began to feel like a combination of Diane Sawyer, Margaret Mead, and Dracula's daughter.

I finally said to him, "I am not your parent or your confessor. You have to decide what all this means to you and bring that to me."

Then Merlin grabbed my hand, "Mommy, race me on the obstacle course!"

It was not an opportune time to process. Later I spotted Oz across the gymnasium, staring down at the floor, looking devastated. I felt so sad for him, but at that moment I decided I had to break up with Oz. We wanted different things in a relationship. It was not worth blowing my family apart or losing Tallulah. Oz needed to go and explore polyamory his way. I needed to find another way to work my life. There was too much instability.

The next evening was our date night. We met at a secluded restaurant.

"It's obvious that you need to date and play the field," I said.

"Are you breaking up with me?" Oz asked.

"I think we need to take a break."

Oz's face crumpled. Tears began to flow down his cheeks, choking sounds came from his throat. Two men at an adjoining table with a pitcher of margaritas glanced at us. I felt a sudden anxiety and also protectiveness of Oz. I thought of Colin Powell's famous Pottery Barn line about invading Iraq: "You break it, you buy it." I was the proud owner of Oz. I felt responsible for him—he'd left his wife. I reached out for his hand. I was surprised (and pleased) by the depth of his attachment to me.

"It's okay, we'll work it out."

Oz calmed down. Back at his apartment, we processed. I assured him I was not breaking up with him, but I couldn't go through the drama anymore or the loss of Tallulah. We made love. Then he said, "I am willing to not date other women, but I want more access to you. I need a domestic partner."

While driving home I thought about how crazy things had gotten and what to do about it. I wasn't sure how to satisfy Oz's needs for domesticity. I thought about the first time Valerie, Oz, Hank, and I had met together to create a unified vision. We had called it a VHOG (Valerie Hank Oz Grace) summit, and we had met way back in March—it was now June. That meeting felt like a lifetime ago. In March, Oz and I had been together just a few weeks. But Oz had suggested we all buy a duplex together. After the meeting, Oz had written an e-mail elaborating more on his vision of how we could cohabitate. It included things like "living communally with Grace and everyone else she loves: Hank, Tallulah, and Merlin," "building a friendship with Hank," and creating "clear boundaries legally, physically, and mentally." Hank was somewhat intrigued but Valerie felt it was way too soon to think of living communally, and the issue was dropped.

Meanwhile, Hank and I were buckling under the humongous cost of our lousy, bloated mortgage, which I'd failed to refinance after the crash of 2008. Oddly enough, just a month before, Hank had come up with the idea to make our large single-family home into a duplex, potentially cutting our costs in half by renting out the other side of the house. In fact, he had already drawn up plans and began what he estimated would be six weeks of noisy, disruptive construction. This was purely financially driven—but I wondered, *Was it possible to revisit the idea of living communally, moving Valerie and Oz in as family?* Although I liked the idea, it felt too soon to bring this up to Hank.

The next afternoon Tallulah and I were having some special time, getting pedicures. We stopped in our favorite boutique to look at clothes. Tallulah tried on some shirts while I spotted a pink lace slip. I imagined modeling it for Oz. I was about to try it on, when suddenly Tallulah was next to me.

"What are you doing?"

I froze, slip in hand.

"Are you going to buy that to wear with Oz?"

"Yes. I mean no—" I started breaking into a sweat.

"Put it back. You are not buying that slip."

"Tallulah, I can buy this slip."

"No. It is inappropriate."

"Tallulah! I am the parent here."

Several people at the boutique looked up. Not because they heard what she said, but because the energy between us was fierce. I was both intimidated and kind of shocked that my kid was lecturing me on appropriate dress.

"You are not buying the slip."

"Tallulah, this is my decision."

This was hardly true. I suddenly felt like I had with my own mother, getting shamed for my needs. Tallulah insisted that we leave—but I had a plan in mind. I walked her to the car, noting with anxiety that she had the swagger of an Aryan youth. I silently unlocked her door. She got inside.

"Okay, honey, I'll be right back."

I was determined to get the damn slip!

"No! You are not going into that store."

"Tallulah, wait in the car!"

"No, that slip is too sexual!"

Did I get to be sexual and a mother at the same time? Was it really so bad to buy lingerie with my ten-year-old daughter? Shaken, I finally folded. I got into the car. Tallulah started ranting about the damn slip. I calmed myself and tried again.

"Tallulah, I am going to take good care of you," I said.

Tallulah snorted.

"You are my priority. I love you and that isn't changing."

"Thanks. That's very reassuring," she replied sarcastically.

Damn! I had said exactly what all the therapists said to say— verbatim. Before kids, when I imagined motherhood, I pictured a series of conversations in which my children's faces would glow at me like I was the Dalai Mama. I never imagined how challenging it would be to meet my needs and theirs at the same time. I was unglued. What kind of a heartless bitch was I? I heard the Mother Mantra: *Suck it up and take care of your kid. It's her turn now; you had yours.*

"Why can't you be like the other mothers? You tried to buy lingerie during our special time!"

"I can buy lingerie."

But now even I wasn't on my side.

"Why can't you go to more PTA meetings?"

Oh, no. Did she just say that? Any energy I had drained away and I was mute. I did support the PTA, dressing as a witch (my own private joke) and giving Tarot readings at the yearly PTA fundraising carnival. My booth had become an almost cultish success with long lines of people coming year after year. I thought I'd mention this to Tallulah.

"My tarot booth supports the PTA."

"Why can't you be the PTA president? Brittany's mother has been the PTA president for three years."

Goddess, I couldn't stand Brittany. That Stepford child with her iPods, laptops, designer clothes, tutors, soccer practice, and private lessons—and her tense workaholic mother, an über–soccer mom driving Brittany to three different events every day after school.

Tallulah raged on. "And you never get the permission slips in on time!"

The damn permission slips! The endless parade of permission slips: to the zoo, the *Nutcracker Suite*, the museum. Every few weeks I had to fill out yet another field trip permission slip. *Just take my kid already! On all your damn field trips—I give you permission!*

Now I fully believed Tallulah: I was a failure as a parent. I was also exhausted. I needed a martini and my date with Oz. And sex. I looked at the clock. It would take seven minutes to get home and another two hours of family time before my date—which I now needed like a drug. I wasn't sure I could make it; my heart was fluttering. I felt even more shame—I wasn't having fun with Tallulah. Looking back at this moment, it amazes me that I expected myself to have fun with someone who was righteously dragging me over the coals.

As I navigated the car through traffic, I suddenly started thinking about my own mother and what it was like to be trapped in a car with her. My mother had frequently shamed me for having any needs that conflicted with her own agenda. After her divorce from Ralph, a smaller personality would have wilted, but my mother vented her outrage on a regular basis.

I remembered a particular October night when my sister was ten, and I was nine. We were sitting on my bed looking out on our street. We had just carved our Halloween pumpkin and placed it on our front vestibule steps. Three teenage boys sauntered up the street, stopped at our pumpkin, then picked it up and smashed it. My sister and I ran yelling for my mother. Moments later I was in the front seat of my mother's car, identifying potential pumpkin attackers. My sister had retreated to her room refusing to get in the vehicle.

We saw some boys walking up Pleasant Street. My mother pulled up next to them, driving slowly at their pace.

"Someone smashed our pumpkin," she said to them.

Oddly, my mother's Boston accent had deepened post-Ralph, almost like a verbal malady that had increased with bitterness, no longer the Cape Cod debutante; she had the vowel slur of a Mack truck driver. The boys looked at her and stifled laughs. One of them called out, "Yeah, lady, we saw your pumpkin."

Taking their statement as a verified confession, my mother pulled her car over the sidewalk, blocking their pathway. She leaned out her window and in her heavy Boston accent barked, "Get in the car! This is a citizen's arrest!" The boys looked at her like her hair had just burst into flames—then they bolted up the street. I begged my mother to go home. I was as frightened as the boys. But she gunned the engine of her Chevy Wagoneer, her tires screeching as she zoomed up the street after them.

The three boys ran up the dead-end cul-de-sac, trapped with their backs against a six-foot-tall fence; they turned just as my mother pulled her station wagon in front of them, her tires wailing as she slammed on the brakes just short of their bodies. Terror rippled across their faces as they realized there was no escape. My mother bellowed, "Get in the car! This is a citizen's arrest!" The "a" in "car" was extended like a ricochet of bullets—JFK with Tourette's syndrome—*caaaaah!*

Two of the boys clawed their way over the fence. The last teenager, trapped, started crying, begging her to not arrest him. I was begging her to go home! My mother got out of the car and sauntered up to the boy, who panicked and dove into a blackberry bush, swam through it into the yard next door, then rolled to the ground and ran away at top speed. My mother watched him go, and then slowly got back in the car. She turned to me with bewilderment, "Do you think we scared them?"

Even in her efforts to protect me, my mother had no clue what a terrifying, destabilizing force she was. *Was I blowing it to the same degree?* A crazy, poly, PTA-defying, hippie mom whom Tallulah would bemoan and dissect in therapy—*just as I had my own mother?* My whole childhood had been chaotic; I was dragged through my mother's crisis-ridden life. As an adult, I had prided myself on breaking my family patterns of instability by creating a happy family with Hank. But was I ruining my family and relationship with Tallulah?

As I steered the car to home with Tallulah pouting in the backseat, I thought about the duplex idea. There just had to be a way to have both—my passion and a stable, loving family—*there just had to be a way.*

Chapter 14

Hank and I sat solemnly in our new therapist's office surrounded by two large ferns. I tried to remember the joke about the therapist with ferns in her office—or was it fern bars? My mind was wandering. I wasn't having fun this therapy go-round. I wasn't sure our therapist had the chops to help us.

Hank commented after our initial introductory session, "How can she coach us on polyamory? She doesn't look like she's had sex in years."

It was true. She didn't look like she'd gotten laid recently. But the pickings of therapists who had empathy for poly parents were mighty slim. She was the only therapist who wasn't smug when I told her our family situation.

After our first session with Tallulah, this therapist suggested we come alone to focus on our marriage. At our second appointment we discussed all the changes going on and how to create more stability for Tallulah. In that session I had pondered my feelings of guilt. I had swallowed the cultural syrup that the main component of a good family was stability. But I knew the one constant in life is change. So I also felt this was our opportunity to coach Tallulah on how to advocate for herself and get what she needed through this transition.

But now in our third session, I was feeling my anxiety mounting again. Hank had just piped up saying that it was time to "turn down the volume" on our special friends and see less of them. I was reminded of the quote from Lao Tzu: "From one comes two, / From two come three, / From the three comes the ten-thousand things." On this third visit it felt like the ten thousand things were about to burst like a rain cloud before a storm.

Hank continued, "We're spending too much time away from home. It's just not working for the kids…."

But I suspected it was really not working for *him*. He wanted me to see less of Oz. We were at a serious juncture.

After yet another long pause, during which I was trying to calculate how much two minutes of silence was costing me at her exorbitant hourly rate, the therapist asked, "Grace, what are you thinking?"

I felt a lead weight pressing down on my chest.

"I just can't imagine seeing less of Oz."

"Well, I think we need to," said Hank. "The kids are beginning to suffer. We are both going away twice a week."

"Isn't there a different way we could do this?"

"I think we need to scale things down and focus on our family."

There was another heavy pause. I felt lava burning at the pit of my stomach. I covered my mouth nervously with my fingers.

"What's going on, Grace?" our therapist asked.

"I am upset."

"Can you tell Hank?"

I took a breath. "When I need you most, you withdraw. You stopped having sex with me when you met Valerie, and then you retracted my overnights with Oz. When I told you how scared I was about money, you kept buying real estate. I am sick of it!"

I had wanted to do money old-school with little debt—now we were overleveraged through real estate investments. From my perspective this was another example of Hank not responding to my needs and concerns.

"I don't see it that way."

"Well I do. All these years, we said watching football was your version of meditation. But that's bullshit! You were watching football while I was doing therapy and meditating and trying to fix myself. We both believed I was the screwball who needed fixing. But you had work to do, too. I wanted to be closer to you and you wouldn't come along for the ride."

I was crying now, choking back tears.

"Now you want me to give up someone who comes through for me. No! I won't do it."

The room was silent except for my heavy breathing. Hank's eyes were cast down on the floor. I felt as if my words had flung him across the room and crushed every bone in his body. I had not wanted to hurt him.

Our therapist informed us we had run over our time. She asked him if he wanted to respond. He said no. She gave us a little reparative speech about "getting to the heart of things" and "this was progress." Then she opened her calendar.

"Shall we book another appointment?"

I looked over at Hank. He turned my way but didn't make eye contact; his body was deflated.

"We'll call you," I mumbled.

Outside, I told Hank I needed time alone. I started to walk what felt like a death march home. Misery was coursing through every vein of my body. Oz called and asked how it all went. I briefly described the carnage.

He listened and then said, "I am so in love with you. Whatever you need I can help you."

Lately it seemed that Oz was pussyfooting around making a traditional commitment. He would say things that implied that whatever happened he wanted to be with me. I clung to his devotion like a lifeline, yet I couldn't dismiss the feeling that he could torque that line at any moment, since he was under tremendous pressure himself. I thanked Oz and told him I would call him back.

Walking down the sidewalk, I had a huge urge to just chuck it all and do it the way everyone else does. Recently, one of my friends had said to me, "You need to get a divorce. You're just too scared to do it." I wondered if that was true. I thought about it as I walked.

The sun was setting. Shattuck Avenue was bustling with people getting off the train, going in and out of the shops, buying food to bring home. Home was the place I had created with Hank. Before Hank, I had felt homeless. Although I was tired of my marriage dynamic with Hank, the traditional divorce scenario seemed like someone else's life. I imagined leaving Hank and seeing my kids half the week. It seemed both terrifying and drastic. I needed my kids in my life every day, and Hank was family. I wanted to raise our kids together. We had weathered so much as a couple, surely there was a way through this.

After walking a good mile, I saw a new waxing shop that advertised hair removal for nearly every square inch that hair could grow on a body. There was a special rate for a Brazilian. I had always wanted to get one—it had been on my Things I'd Like To Try list for years. This was the day. Once, in my twenties when I was depressed, I cut off my long hair. A crew cut seemed like the jolt that I needed. Getting waxed felt similar but more painful. It was like electric shock for the pussy—the physical pain made me feel more in control of my life. I was a tough girl—a female Clint Eastwood saying, "Go ahead, wax my pussy!" *Yeah, I could handle whatever life dished out.* When it was done I felt renewed.

I didn't want everything to spin out of control. I wanted us all to get our needs met. The duplex idea popped into my head again. *Was there a way to cohabitate?*

When I got home Hank was in the backyard, which was littered with lumber, paint cans, and tools. He sat smoking in a lawn chair. His eyes looked startled. I felt immensely sad. I wanted him to know I was still bonded to him, but the fact was his worst nightmare had happened and we could both feel it. Oz had become a primary relationship to me. I had not anticipated this happening, and at the time I felt too guilty to admit that perhaps I had been searching for this. Part of doing poly was to set Hank up with a nice gal so I could avoid hurting him. I was like one of those heroines in the movies who fixes up her husband before she dies—minus the terminal illness. The reality had been brewing for a long time: I needed more from Hank. Whether we were doing poly or monogamy, this was the truth.

After our catastrophic therapy session, Hank went full speed on the duplex conversion. It was clearly a response to my anger over our financial vulnerability. It was 2010, two years after the banks had been bailed out. There were so many reports of foreclosures in the news that I was scared we might be next if we did not make drastic changes.

The weekend after the therapy session, Hank, the kids, and I drove to Palm Springs to visit old friends. It was a relief to be with friends we'd known for decades but who had no idea about the current turmoil in our lives. We talked about our work, our children, the weather—we didn't dare discuss the tectonic plates of chaos and uncertainty that were shifting beneath our feet.

During our first dinner together, the wife asked me to help her husband with his knees. Having watched this man walk earlier, I already knew which muscles were tight and which were weak. The husband's voice took on a steely quality as he said that he'd book a session back home at my studio. To which the wife replied, "Never going to happen. Never." Then things got particularly tense. I'd experienced this phenomenon before: a simple squabble between spouses about how to approach a problem, escalating into a massive argument about something much, much more than the muscular health of a body part. Once again, I became witness to a hint of what were undoubtedly years of anger bubbling up, fossilized, and cemented over with regret and compromises. Their voices got quieter, which made their heated debate feel more chilling. Mesmerized, I watched them, my heart beating nervously. This was the long-married hostile couple I had feared we would become.

My trance was broken by Tallulah climbing into my lap. Pulling her close, I felt her breath start to regulate as she leaned into my chest. She was my vibes keeper, my little witch, so aware of everything around her. I thought it must be frightening for her to watch this couple's discord. Then suddenly I became viscerally aware that she must be witnessing the transformation of my marriage with Hank. I began to imagine how unnerving that must be for her.

I started to sing very softly into her ear. Her body eased as I stroked her hair. I began to recall those first days after discovering I was pregnant with Tallulah, when I felt an almost crushing responsibility for the separate being who was growing in my body. A maternal stress developed, which surely contributed to a pregnancy-induced ass swell that defied science—my hemorrhoids made morning sickness look glamorous. I had a home birth that happened with the speed of a freight train, three short hours start to finish. When it was time to push, I was helped up onto the birthing stool, a hollow chair with an open seat. I've always been a pusher, trying to hasten everything with my supreme drive to keep going, my witchy mentors chiding me, "Don't try to push the river." But this was my moment, and like a confident pinch hitter called in to close the game, I breathed in, then with one massive push Tallulah came flying down the birth canal.

The midwife literally scrambled to catch Tallulah, who was then lifted up to my arms. I'd done magic to have a fast birth (so afraid of the potential pain), and *Goddess had it worked!* I'd made a pact with Tallulah: she could pick the time, but once she started that first contraction—*go straight for the door, burrow out*—pronto!

As I held my daughter in those first moments of meeting her, I was awestruck by this intelligent being—who had heard every one of my requests *and responded with mastery.* I was also moved by her tiny vulnerability—and her complete dependence on me. As I held her tightly against my chest—her wiry, slippery limbs wet from birth and my whole body shaking post-delivery—I could feel the stress and fear of motherhood begin to ease as I was transported into a whole new view of the role. I was helped to our queen bed to breastfeed. As Tallulah suckled, I was overcome by a feeling I'd never had as a kid—a grounded solidity. I was Tallulah's home base—it was an experience that I had not received as a child; now I was the source of it.

I looked around the table; the couple was silently serving dessert. Merlin played with a deck of cards next to Hank, who was staring off into space. I tried to catch Hank's eye. But I wasn't sure he'd even fully registered the depth of the fight we'd just witnessed. He sipped his drink and looked as if he were designing architecture at a drafting table in the sky. Tallulah sighed, then nestled closer into my body. I could feel she was in a better state now. Tallulah knew everything; this was an overwhelming fact. All kids knew whether their parents were happy or sad—perhaps they were not fully conscious of it, but they knew.

At that moment it occurred to me how much Tallulah needed me to make it safe. I was her mama, I was the Earth. Maybe Hank was the Sun and the sky, but you depended on Earth to cradle you.

After dinner, while getting ready for bed, Hank told me that Valerie was beyond angry. She felt excluded and deeply wounded that he had not at least told his friends about her. The next day I exchanged several texts with Oz, who also felt excluded from the family vacation. When we got home, Hank approached me in the kitchen after we had put the kids to bed. He told me Valerie had tried to break up with him but he convinced her to hang on.

Seeing our lovers twice a week on the side was not working. I had not anticipated this when we started doing poly. Somehow I imagined our secondary partners as chipper and satisfied. The poly books talked about people who did not want family life, who wanted more time to themselves—these were people who wanted to be secondary partners. But Oz and Valerie wanted more.

A few days later, I had a date with Oz. After we made love we languished in his apartment in yet another state of postcoital bliss. I was writing on my laptop. Oz looked up at me with those luscious seafoam green eyes and said, "I want to hear what you've written in your journal."

"It's nothing that interesting."

"But I want to hear what you are thinking. I want to know everything about you—you fascinate me."

I loved that Oz was so interested in me as a writer, an artist, a woman.

I had been musing on what it felt like to have two men in my life. One man represented family and stability, the other a hot spicy roll in the hay. I liked Oz's penthouse and the division of my life: how when I arrived it was all about sex and conversation; no one asking me to do the dishes or pay the phone bill, our biggest consternation being the timing of orgasm. Meeting up with Oz—but not living together—was like getting a hermetically sealed dose of romance and sex. So I had been journaling about male entitlement around sexual pleasure and toying with the idea of a woman getting to have the same. I was exploring what it meant for her relationships if she did.

So without much further thought I read him the full page. Afterward, a silence came over the room.

"Are you okay?" I asked Oz.

"Yes," he replied, but his face was contorted with pain.

"What's going on?"

"Is that what I am to you? A piece of ass? Your excitement on the side?"

"No! No, not at all."

Oz went out on the balcony. I followed him. He was too choked up to talk. He looked up at the sky, then tears streamed down his face.

"This situation is untenable. I will hold on as long as I can, but I can't do it much longer."

Oz was crying *again*. *Wow*, the thought popped into my head unbridled, *he's such a girl*. I liked that he was in touch with his feminine side—and yet, he was a reminder of a short affair I'd had with a dancer in New York City. The sex was amazing, but every once in a while she'd get emotional over her orgasm or mine—and then we'd wind up spending hours discussing her feelings.

Sometimes Oz felt like the same kind of drama queen. I wanted to wail, *I got mine—get yours*, the famous lament coined by Richard Pryor. It seemed like Oz was laying his whole life at my feet, and I was supposed to make it all right with a big orgasmic bow. It was an unfair responsibility, the weight of which I only felt for my children.

"I want a domestic partner too," he said.

We stood facing each other on the balcony with its views of the bay, the Golden Gate Bridge, and fog-engulfed San Francisco. Oz had been given so much privilege—couldn't he hang tough for a few months till we sorted this all out? I just didn't get it. But Oz kept crying. I went over and took his hand.

"Baby, it's okay. I want you, too."

"Do you? Because I want a solid family, too."

I was silent. The truth was, although Oz was my best ride, he was one scary pony to bet on. One minute he was declaring his everlasting love and the next he was saying, "But I may have to sleep with other women!" I didn't want to move Oz into my home and then find out that he *just had to move in* his new favorite girlfriend as well. I felt protective of myself and my kids. I was sure we could create some openness in our relationship over time, but I feared he might be like the shallow poly man-hos with a sprinkling of seductive emotional angst veiling his narcissism.

Oz continued, "I—I don't want to break the poly rules, and I don't want you and Hank to go through the agony of a divorce like me but, but—"

"What?"

"I want you to be my family. I want to grow old with you."

I came up to him and reached for his hand. Oz grabbed me in a big bear hug. There was a dire quality to his grasp, which still baffled me. He was a good guy, but was it right to have him move in? How would I ever propose this to Hank?

In all the uncertainty, one thing was very certain: to maintain financial stability we needed to rent out one side of our soon-to-be duplex as soon as construction was over in two weeks. I had to clean out all of our rooms and get rid of half of my stuff, which seemed like the perfect metaphor for my life at the time: let go of the superfluous. I hired Vivi, my clutter-clearing gal. She arrived early morning, and when I described the massive task at hand, she seemed to understand empirically that we were not only cleaning out half our rooms—we were cleaning out karma. I loved her emboldened style, jumping in with no hesitation, holding up items, and interrogating me like a cop: "Do you use it? Do you need it? When was the last time you touched it?"

We tossed half my makeup collection, Vivi acting with the heartlessness of the Khmer Rouge as she held up an impulsive Sephora purchase of glitter tanning gel.

"Really?" she teased. "When was the last time you used this?"

We ditched some garish sunglasses from a trip to Las Vegas, for which Hank's great-aunt had given us hundred dollar bills to go on a shopping splurge. Later, looking at our purchases in the hotel room, Hank had said, "Isn't it odd how shopping makes you feel like you really accomplished something?" It always had, the material goods filling one with the heady experience of prosperity. But I remembered an old witch saying to me, when I was making a trea-sure map to manifest prosperity, "You do realize prosperity is so much more than having money?"

After clutter clearing the entire downstairs, progress suddenly stalled at my upstairs bedroom closet, where I had stashed dozens and dozens of snapshots of Tallulah and Merlin as babies, toddlers—first days of school, trips to the zoo. I found a picture of me and Tallulah making a homemade pizza; I was nine months pregnant with Merlin, opulent with life and due any minute. I clutched the photo, anxiously trying to decide which pictures to keep and which to throw away. It was becoming a photographic *Sophie's Choice*, when Vivi gently took the pile of photos from my hands.

"Here," she said, placing them in a large box on my bed, "You get to have all of them. You don't have to choose," she said quietly.

I sat on the bed, embarrassed by my emotionality as relief flooded over me. I stared at a photo of me pregnant with Merlin, in the last months of my pregnancy, so joyous that I had carried my baby to term.

When Tallulah was two years old, I started trying to get preg-nant again. The first miscarriage came quickly. The doctors called it a "blighted ovum." I called all my friends, sobbing over my blighted ovum, until Hank said quietly, "Just because they call it a blighted ovum doesn't mean we have to. *We lost our baby.*"

A battery of fertility tests, consultations with a fertility doctor, and several months of deliberation finally led us to decide on IVF. After implanting the embryos, my doctor took my hand solemnly and said, "It's in God's hands now." I thought, *Fuck God, I just paid you ten grand!* The IVF failed, and during the next two years I had two more miscarriages and another IVF.

After my second IVF, I was so jacked up on fertility drugs that I wanted to crawl out of my own skin. I went into an almost cataclys-mic depression when I saw the spots of blood that started my third miscarriage. I felt betrayed by Goddess. But what I couldn't see at the time was that I had betrayed her by sublimating my own body and intuition.

Just days after that final miscarriage I started calling adoption centers, but Hank asked that we wait six months, to grieve. Putting aside my dream for a second child felt like being dragged from the classroom of life and forced to wait patiently in the detention center—letting go is the last and most difficult step in spell work. Even though releasing the outcome had always produced miracles for me, I found it excruciating to let go and let Goddess add her magic.

Six months later we were signed up at an adoption center. I had finally relinquished the idea of a biological child and was now elated about adopting. But the ultimate mastery of spell work asks that we show up and do *everything possible* and then turn over the results. Pondering this challenge, I had asked myself, *Could I try to conceive a baby, while at the same time turning the results over to the Universe?* In that fifth month, when I knew I was ovulating, I seduced Hank three nights in a row. It was more an exercise in surrender, because the doctors had convinced me I had an "ovarian reserve problem"—a clinical way of informing me I was over the fertility hill at forty-two.

Two weeks later I was utterly stunned as I stared at the pregnancy stick. *Goddess had given me my baby!* I could feel the placenta growing as the progesterone suppositories I'd learned about from other infertile mothers in my support group did their job. Every day of my pregnancy with Merlin I woke up feeling like I had won the lottery. I named him Merlin because the wisdom accrued from my fertility odyssey was as powerful as King Arthur's feat of pulling the sword from the stone.

In my need to control nature, I had stopped listening to my own wisdom. And I had also neglected the great feat of burning off all of my mother's negativity about children. At the beginning of my odyssey I was scared I would lose myself with another child. My mother had blamed her failings on her children, angry rants starting with "If I hadn't had you kids—" One night, a year into my odyssey of trying to birth a second child, Hank said, "Isn't it odd that your mother used to say things like that, when you and your brother and sister were the only people who truly loved and took care of her?"

In those two years, it became crystal clear what a gift a baby was. I didn't care anymore if I got fat or sick or my career slowed down for a time. I didn't even care that in my efforts to conceive Merlin I took medication that caused an anal abscess—and if that wasn't humiliating enough, all the doctors at the colorectal department were gorgeous male residents in their twenties with moony eyes and polite smiles, all examining my ass! Throughout nine operations! But the Universe had me on a crash course confronting the wounds and shame from my childhood. I moved on from the surgeries, which had significantly cleaned up the wound, to the unavoidable next piece that required me literally sitting with myself—soaking my behind in daily sitz baths of Chinese herbs while meditating on the years of disowned grief that floated up in the cathartic stillness. I became determined to reclaim the potential gifts of my root chakra—internal security and creating a successful family. If the path to my root chakra was blocked—and I was certain it was—I had to find a way to open it up, allowing the energy and wisdom of my body to flow. In the end, it was the simple act of literally *sitting* with the suppressed emotions I had inherited from both parents that was the final last step that likely healed the abscess—and I had a new sense of myself. I banished my mother's negativity, replacing it with the solid knowledge that I was a different woman: strong, stable, and able to not only grow a baby but to grow a solid home base for my family. Boxing up all my photos, I realized it was all okay as long as I got to have my kids, my family, the memories, the unbroken connection. Everything else was disposable.

That night I sat down with Hank.

"I feel like Oz and Valerie have become family to us—chosen family. I just can't imagine scaling it all down. I need this new life that they are bringing us."

Hank nodded. He had always been a man of few words. It was also true that we were both reluctant to directly address the massive shifts happening in our relationship. I felt as if I were unexpectedly pregnant—now a new life was growing. It was clear to me that Hank needed to digest this and make the next move—whatever that would be.

On the day he secured the last bolt on the circular staircase, we put a bottle of champagne in the refrigerator to chill, then took a walk in the hills.

Hank had a quiet, happy buzz about him.

"What's up?" I asked.

"I've been thinking a lot about our situation."

"Oh, yeah?"

"What if Valerie lived on the new side with me? You and Oz lived on the other side?"

"Say more."

It felt like a delicate moment. I had not asked Hank for this directly. If it was going to happen, he had to come to it himself. Hank continued.

"It doesn't work for both of us to leave twice a week for dates. The kids miss us. It's not sustainable. Valerie feels resentful and secondary. I asked Valerie if she'd be interested in moving in. I wanted to check in with her before suggesting the idea to you."

I nodded, "So Valerie wants to move in?"

"Yes, she loves the kids and she wants to live with me."

"Would you be willing to sit down with Oz and discuss what it would all look like?"

"Yes. I think that would be a good idea. Valerie is concerned about her privacy. She wants locks on the doors so she can have her own space."

"But the kids can go freely back and forth between us?"

I was concerned about what it would be like for Valerie to live with our kids around.

Hank stopped on the wooded trail and turned to me.

"I could never be on this journey with anyone but you," he said.

We hugged. I was thrilled. Somehow we were going through this massive change in our relationship and still loving each other. For me, this was the most significant part of the poly philosophy: adding new people in without losing the love you already had. And I had fought hard for the addition of our new chosen family; I did not want to abort this new life. But what I didn't foresee at the time—and what both of us were unwilling to acknowledge—was how this would change the very structure of our connection. This new beginning would be the end of something between Hank and me, something that perhaps had started to fade years prior. At this moment I was focused on the new life. I didn't want to recognize that, with this passage, an old way of being would also pass. Because, right then, the passage was the revitalization that I needed and was fighting for.

That night I met Oz for dinner. I had told him I had a big surprise for him. He arrived ten minutes after I did—immediately demanding to hear the news.

"How would you like to live in the duplex with me?"

He didn't say anything but his eyes got soft as he gazed at me.

"Baby," I asked, "how are you feeling?"

"I feel great," he said.

I reached across the table, took his hand, and playfully bit his knuckle. "Be careful what you wish for," I said.

"What could you possibly mean? It's always been my life ambition to move in with a nice girl and her husband."

That night, wrapped around each other, Oz whispered in my ear, "When we live together I am going to make love to you every day."

Then he told me that he had a present for me. I thought it might be a diamond, so I sat up in bed. I was flushed with excitement as I tore open the sparkly tissue paper. Then I saw it—a *huge* penis-shaped dildo. We both laughed. I pulled it out of the bag. It was the size of a small rolling pin. It was so large it looked like it was made to scare someone.

"That is mammoth."

"It's the same size as my cock."

"No! It is not the size of your cock."

But O obliged me by pulling out his almost fully erect member then putting the dildo next to it and, sure enough—same size.

"Well, I'll be a monkey's uncle!"

"You said you miss me when I'm gone!"

"But can it solve technical problems on my computer?"

"Its head isn't *that* big."

During the next few days I was giddy with triumph over our new living arrangement. I called all my friends to share the news. But when I started to tell people what we were doing, they responded with alarm. Two friends told me to hire a lawyer to make everything legal and binding. I wondered what they thought Oz and Valerie would do—steal our cutlery? I decided to fly under the radar for a while. I was steadfast in my ideal that we could add in people without losing anyone. But there was still one more hurdle I had to leap over before moving Oz and Valerie in. I was confident in my beliefs as long as I didn't have to explain them to Tallulah. I anticipated telling her of Oz's imminent move-in as one might anticipate a root canal. Freya coached me to present with confidence. The problem was that I was still trying to gain Tallulah's approval. She represented my worst fears. *Was it better to be a selfless, sex-deprived mother and just put all your life energy into your kids?*

I thought again about my own mother. Before the signature on her divorce papers was signed, my mother had gained an insular forty pounds of protective girth. She stayed fat but longed to be thin throughout the rest of my childhood and adolescence, rehashing tales of being sought after by a multitude of beaus. As teenagers, my sister and I asked to inherit her '50s pencil skirts for a costume party.

"You won't fit into those skirts," she said, scanning our bodies like a boxer eyeing her opponent in the ring. "My waist was twenty-five inches back then," she said bitterly. My sister and I would roll our eyes, mesmerized by her wounded and obvious attempts to outdo us.

These stories made my heart ache for her. I vowed that when I became a mother, I would be responsible for my own happiness. I did not want my children burdened with an unhappy mother. I created a situation in which I could satisfy my needs for a lover and keep our family intact—but Tallulah was informing me I was doing it all wrong. My instincts told me she was a kid that needed to be guided through this. If I didn't make these changes I was at risk of being bitter like my mother. In an odd way, what I needed from Tallulah was the approval I had never received from my mentally unstable mother. If I continued to seek Tallulah's approval as if she were the adult in charge, this situation would never work.

It had been a week since we had decided to move Valerie and Oz in. Hank and I had decided to have a conversation with Tallulah in a few more days, on a weekend, when we had more time to spend with her. But Tallulah had sensed a change in the air. Driving home from an afternoon outing with just the two of us, she confronted me.

"Are you planning to move Oz in?"

"We'll discuss it tonight with Daddy," I said.

"He is not moving in!" Tallulah screamed, and then she demanded to know my plans.

I was weary. We drove in silence.

Tallulah screamed again, "Are you trying to move Oz in? He is not moving in!" She kept yelling, "Oz is not moving in!"

I calmly told her to please wait till we got home, but she was in a tantrum.

Finally I yelled, "Yes! Okay, yes! Oz is moving in."

Tallulah let out an enraged howl, but this time I howled back. *Damn, there goes the Mother of the Year award,* I thought to myself.

When we got home, she ran upstairs and slammed her bedroom door so hard I thought it would crack. I opened it and willed myself to take the tone of an adult in charge.

"Tallulah," I began, "the decision is not yours to make. I will continue to do everything possible to help you through this transition. But I am done with this discussion. Oz is a good person or I would not let him move in. I am willing to do everything to help you thrive. But I will not give up my happiness for you."

What happened next shocked both of us: she calmed down. Her rigid little being relaxed, and she looked up at me with eyes that needed reassurance. I stood confused, almost like the tornado had leaped over my house and was now evaporating into the clouds. It was unexpected.

She mumbled, "Okay, Mommy."

Then she sat down on the bed with exhaustion. I went to her and wrapped my arm around her waist. Her head fell on my shoulder.

"What's going on, baby?"

"I just want it to be the four of us. I don't want that to change."

There were so many things about our life that Tallulah did not know, and I was not about to tell her. I needed things to change. If they didn't, I imagined myself a bitter raging version of my mother. I was steering our lives, confident that in the long run we were heading to a good place.

"I understand. It must feel scary to you."

Tallulah nodded, a tear trickled down her cheek.

"Oh, my love." I rubbed her back. "Baby, a lot is changing. It's true, but there's one thing that's not changing. I love you so much. You and Merlin are the most important thing for me. I am thinking of you both."

"Okay, Mommy," Tallulah yawned, then crawled into my lap. I rocked her silently for many minutes.

"Mommy, I love it when you hold me."

"I love it too, sweetie."

We decided to watch a movie. I made popcorn and we snuggled together.

After Tallulah fell asleep, I called Freya to report the day's happening. Freya volunteered to explain to Tallulah how she does family. We decided to meet for lunch the next day. When we sat down, Freya started explaining how she still lives with her former husband. They divorced years ago, but are still family. When Freya discovered that she was a lesbian, he had helped her come out. Freya's voice was like velvet. I sank back into my chair, sipping my Cabernet. Tallulah asked Freya a multitude of questions. I could see her ten-year-old brain expanding past the "normal" family setup.

At one point she said, "I like Oz, I just don't like poly."

"What is it that you don't like?" I asked.

"None of my friends' parents are doing this. I'm embarrassed. I also don't want Daddy to go away."

I reassured her that it was our intention to stay close.

On the walk home, Tallulah asked, "Do you love Daddy?"

"Sweetie, I've known Daddy for twenty-five years. We grew each other up. I love him very much. He's my people."

"Do others have family like this?

"I don't know of many who are doing it like we are."

"Why?"

"I am not sure. Everyone has their own way of doing things. It is more common in the gay community to stay close to partners as the relationship changes."

"It is so scary for me if you stop loving Daddy."

Tallulah stopped on the sidewalk, softly crying. I pulled her close to me.

"It's okay, my love, it will be okay. I'll make sure of it."

When we got back to the house Hank was making marinara sauce, while Merlin sat on Valerie's lap. Hank offered me a taste of the sauce. It was a recipe my father had given Hank nearly twenty years ago on a visit—which had turned out to be another failed attempt to create a father-daughter relationship. When my parents divorced I was a baby. At six I had asked my mother if I could meet my father. I remember a handful of visits in which my mother stood seething in the corner while I sat on my stepmother Angela's lap. My father had left my mother to be with Angela, his former girlfriend from the Bronx. I actually liked Angela. She gave me butterscotch lifesavers from her purse and told me I was lovely, but I quickly stopped gravitating to her after my mother pulled me into a corner and hissed, "Never sit on Angela's lap again!"

Tallulah asked Valerie if she could paint Valerie's fingernails, then ran off to get her manicure gear. I sat down next to Valerie and Merlin. I started chatting with Valerie as I playfully took Merlin's feet into my lap. The whole idea was to have more love, not less like what happened to me as a child. What we were doing was good. I felt this in my bones. Hank carried a large bowl of pasta to the table; I decided to indulge. We passed around the vermicelli then the marinara sauce. For the first time in a long while, I felt like everything was going to be okay.

Chapter 15

Tallulah and I were at our favorite box store buying "designer labels for less!" We were picking out new sheets for our bedrooms. Tallulah picked up a set of purple sheets.

"Look, Mom, 500 thread count!"

Someone had ripped open the package; we touched the silky material.

"Very nice."

"Can I get them?"

"Sure."

I had offered to totally redecorate Tallulah's bedroom with her. It was part fun-project and part positive-distraction-while-I-quietly-move-Oz-in. I grabbed some silk bedding for me and Oz. I imagined us between the sheets—in our new bedroom.

"Are you getting those for you?"

"Yes," I said a bit apprehensively.

I was purposely steering clear of any discussion of my new bed with Oz. I could play the role of the docile PTA mother for a few hours—while illicitly buying silk sheets for me and my lover.

Valerie had already slept over a few nights on Hank's side of the house and had seamlessly been accepted by Tallulah. But there was a clear double standard where Oz and I were concerned. It was that mother prejudice again—it was all okay if Mommy was knitting in the back room, but I clearly wouldn't be knitting with Oz.

As a woman, Valerie represented nurture and was therefore unthreatening, but Oz represented me being sexual. In Tallulah's mind, adding in a man meant less nurturing for her. But I knew this wouldn't be true. There were several nights when Oz had been hanging out and spontaneously started helping Tallulah with her homework. He would nurture her too. If I hadn't been sure of this, I would not have wanted him to move in.

Tallulah wasn't the only one adjusting; it was still a stretch for Hank to allow Oz to move in. I could see he was happy for Valerie to be in-house—that was good for him—but I could feel his brain clicking over to the fact that this meant I got to have Oz as well. I knew Hank did not fully accept my love for Oz. I didn't know what to do about that, so I did nothing. My main strategy the last few weeks after we'd hit the impasse in therapy was to meditate, pray, and get my pussy waxed. All the great traditions of spirituality frequently advise that you do nothing. In this case it worked for me.

But I was keenly aware of Hank's pain. I felt self-conscious—even ashamed—about feeling so good about Oz and the changes in our family. I had an almost metallic urgency to want Hank to be happy. When I would update my friends on our situation, I would gloss over any grief, putting a newfangled Brady Bunch twist on things. I was stumped as to how to help Hank's suffering. Hank and I had always been comrades in our pain, he with his Holocaust background, me with the violence from my childhood. Hank and I understood the angst of the survivors, the ambivalence of being the one who made it.

My sister had never recovered from what we survived as kids with Ralph. She'd had several emotional breakdowns and lived largely in an imaginary world. Once, when my sister visited Hank and me, she manically talked about her upcoming lunch date with Rose Kennedy, who had been dead for years. Hank smiled at her, then whimsically said, "Rose Kennedy, huh? I've always wanted to meet her." He knew instinctively her psyche was latching on to a famous family and trying to help her nurse herself to a better place.

But now I was having survivor's guilt—around Hank. For years I'd been nursing myself to a better place, taking small steps every day, learning to soothe my nervous system. These baby steps had amassed, putting me in a lighter, more expansive place. I had wanted

Hank to join me in this new place. But I was beginning to recognize that the accumulation of each little step had put significant distance between us. Distance that I was only realizing now at this juncture. Hank was still occupying a land I knew only too well, a place where you hold heavy despair as a loyalty to those who had not made it.

I would never forget those I lost—not a day went by that my sister in particular was not present in my thoughts. But I had a new way to be loyal to her. What if a person had gained the capacity to be fuller and stronger, with more energy to give? I was partially embarrassed to be here—I felt cloaked and even conflicted about it. But it was my children who most inspired me. I knew what it was to have pain handed down to you, tight knots that you had to untangle on your own. I wanted my children to be empathic to suffering but also have an energetic inheritance, an innate entitlement to create great lives for themselves, for me, for the world. I wasn't helping my sister when I overate on the Toll House cookies we used to bake together as kids; I was helping her by living a bigger life that hopefully I could pull her into. The more people who evolve, the better it is for everyone—even beyond the scope of my family.

But was I losing Hank in the process? This was devastating to contemplate. I was hoping that Valerie could help Hank, although I felt remorse passing the torch to her. Shouldn't I have been able to pull him into a better place? I continued to be the movie-heroine-minus-the-terminal-illness making sure her husband was good so I could go off and not die but actually live it up.

I put all my efforts into making our new situation work. Whatever Valerie needed I eagerly accommodated. Oz and Valerie were giving us a huge gift by allowing us to keep our family intact. Oz was very vocal about how much he supported this living arrangement; he knew as a parent what it meant.

He would say to me, "You're getting everything you wanted—your kids, my love, and Hank's love. I am so impressed with you."

I was so impressed that Oz could be so emotionally generous, when I knew that it was bittersweet for him. He had wanted the same thing for himself: to be able to see his kids every day and to have a loving co-parenting situation.

Two weeks after Hank's decision to let Oz and Valerie move in, Oz came over to watch a football game with Hank. Yes, it was a cliché, but I was so happy that I made snacks for them. Hank was contained but friendly. Over the past four years, Hank had never put Oz down and several times had made clear his empathy for Oz, but I wasn't sure how he was feeling now. Hank and I had been through a lot around our marriage and in particular my attraction to Oz, and he kept most of his emotions to himself. But it seemed to me that their bro time that afternoon was a good sign. Maybe Hank was starting to realize that Oz was not competing with him.

After the football game, Oz and Hank went off to a café to discuss the living arrangement. Hank told me later that he had made a sketch of both sides of the house. Hank proposed that he and Valerie live on the new side, which had the feel of a townhouse. It was connected to what would be my side of the house through two doors, one on each floor: Downstairs, a door in my dining room would lead into their kitchen. Up a spiral staircase on the townhouse side, a door would connect their living room to my hallway, which led to Tallulah and Merlin's bedrooms. I was excited that the kids could easily travel back and forth from Hank and me on both floors. There would be no community spaces except for the large lawn, which both of our side doors led into.

Hank and Oz discussed how to set up the kids in their respective bedrooms. They went through several scenarios, then decided that Merlin and Liam (because they were so excited to) would share a bedroom, and the girls would each have their own separate rooms.

I could have gone to the meeting but instead sat home holding my breath. I knew this was a moment that required me to step back. Hank and Oz needed to work out the delicate balance of their relationship. Under these circumstances, even liking each other was unprecedented. There were cultural categories for women who cohabit with men—harem sisters, polygamous wives, et cetera (not that these were models for me and Valerie)—but where in history did you ever see two boys making it work for the woman they both loved?

I wanted everyone to love each other and be supremely happy—because I was supremely happy. I was scared that somehow, because, as Oz said, I got everything I wanted, I was going to be perceived as selfish, a narcissist controlling "my two men." I ran my fear by one of my poly friends. We discussed how these stereotypes were embedded in all of us. In the media, the movies, and in our art and politics was this notion that somehow being multipartnered was connected to cheating and exploitation. Having a good guy and a bad guy seemed essential to every story, plot, or artwork. I realized I had to clean up my own thinking. I had internalized this dichotomy. It was fine to have two men in my life, and we were all creating this situation together—even though people might assume otherwise.

Hank suggested we start doing VHOGs again to prepare for "officially" moving Oz and Valerie in, since they were sleeping over more regularly anyway. Tallulah requested to speak at a summit. She was pissed off when Hank and I would occasionally sleep over at Valerie or Oz's apartments. As the eldest child, Tallulah was taking on a role of a small senator.

She said, "I feel afraid when I suddenly hear that Daddy is going to Valerie's house for the night, or you are going to Oz's apartment. I want to know ahead of time."

She wanted a clear schedule with a week's notice of who would be leaving the house and when.

My hopes were to build a home in which children's and parents' needs were balanced. If Valerie and Oz moved in full-time, it would solve the problem of Hank and I leaving the kids overnight. Watching Tallulah express herself so confidently made me feel that we must be doing something right. I was still attending counseling sessions with Tallulah and Judy. In one session Tallulah talked about how she really liked Valerie and Oz. But she said that she'd feel better if more people were doing poly. Judy explained how about thirty years ago Hank and I getting married would have been a huge deal, since Hank is Jewish and I was raised Christian. Then Judy discussed interracial marriages—how they used to be illegal and how gay marriages still are in many places. Just twenty years ago it was unheard of to have two mommies. Now it was socially acceptable, at least in the Bay Area, to have same-gendered parents.

These discussions helped Tallulah, but she had developed a fear that Hank would leave the house when I was on a date night with Oz. Tallulah sensed the vast changes in my relationship with Hank. She could feel me aligning more with Oz. This made her worry about losing Hank. One night, returning from my date, I came to kiss Tallulah good night. She was anxiously crying in bed. I cradled her in my arms and called out to Hank who came and sat close by.

"Honey, I would never leave you alone. Have I ever done anything like that?" Hank asked.

Tallulah agreed that no, he had not. After I tucked her back in bed, I talked to Hank about it. We acknowledged that her fears were about all the changes in our lives. We decided to find her a child therapist so she could work out her anxiety in a more conscious way. Our model was the poly model of addition and not subtraction of people; but we were in a huge state of flux, and all she saw around her was the divorce model, which usually means that someone leaves.

At the VHOGs we discussed the kids extensively, sharing insights and information about how they were adjusting. We also discussed how each of the adults was adjusting. Part of our manifesto was to honor each person's experience. We would do an emotional check-in for the first part of the VHOG. At one meeting Hank put on the agenda that he wanted to "support Valerie to express her needs," and he gently urged her to share what was present for her.

Valerie said she "got triggered" at the last summit when Oz and I were "very physically affectionate." I had given Oz a foot massage as we talked. She admitted that she may have been longing for the same kind of attention from Hank because they had had a spat before the meeting. Nevertheless, it made her uncomfortable. So we discussed how to handle physical affection in each other's presence. I reassured Valerie that I wasn't triggered by any affection between her and Hank. We were operating as two couples now. We did not share information about our agreements between each other, but both Valerie and Oz had told me they'd be okay with it if I wanted to sleep with Hank. I was sort of suspicious of their generosity, given the dormant state of my sex life with Hank.

I'd like to say that Hank and I sat down and had a thorough discussion about our agreements, but we did not. Hank and I did not make conscious agreements at this time because we both sensed that this would be too hard, and, for the first time in decades, I—who could have out-processed Freud—was not interested in discussing it. I assumed we were both kind of on the same page, which was that sex between us had become an effort, and we had let it go. I thought this was how Hank felt too, until Valerie's light box exhibition.

The night of the exhibition, Oz and I arrived at the San Francisco gallery about an hour after it all started. The energy was high. Valerie, Hank, Tallulah, and Merlin had arrived much earlier to set things up. Tallulah and Merlin were wearing illuminated light boxes around their torsos and serving hors d'oeuvres to lots of hipsters dressed to the nines. I started making my way around the room, chatting it up with Valerie's friends.

After an hour, I signaled to Oz that it was time to hit the open road. It was our date night and I wanted to take him to a bar two blocks away that I used to hang at with all my actor pals. A little tipsy, I went over to Hank and kissed him on the lips good-bye. Then I went to get my jacket in the coatroom. When I turned around Hank was beside me. I assumed he was going to give me a kid report, but instead he leaned in and kissed me. *A real kiss.* I was stunned. Then Oz walked in to get his coat. There was a little tension in the air.

"Hello," Oz said.

"Hi," I blurted like a frog.

I felt like I was cheating on my lover with my husband. So far this had not been an issue, so Oz and I had no real agreements (e.g., Yes, Grace may occasionally tongue-kiss Hank). We said our good-byes, then Oz and I stepped out into the cool night. Several people stood at the entrance to the loft, smoking. I could see the neon sign to the bar I wanted to take Oz to. It was flashing the outline of a martini glass. I leaned into Oz as we walked.

"Now that we'll be living together soon," Oz said, "and I feel we are a couple, I feel oddly jealous. Did you kiss Hank?"

"I guess. I... I..." I was flustered.

"I don't know how I'd feel if you slept with Hank. I think I'd be okay with it."

"I don't think that's going to happen."

I didn't really want it to happen. In fact, the whole kissing episode had made me feel oddly embarrassed. We went to the bar and talked some more about our agreements. Oz was fascinated by my relationship to Hank. He stated again how much he wanted to support our love. I told him I was sure this was an isolated drunken incident.

That night when we got back to Oz's penthouse, with much reluctance and embarrassment I described to Oz a porn video I'd masturbated over that very afternoon.

"Let's watch it together!" he immediately suggested.

"I don't know," I said.

Oz pulled out his laptop and started searching for the video. *What was I afraid of?* I was afraid he'd be turned on by the politically incorrect video.

We started watching it.

"Stop," I said, "It's too scary. I'll just hate you if you get turned on."

Oz laughed.

"No, it isn't funny."

"So I am not allowed to get turned on by it but you can?"

"The things that turn me on sometimes disturb me. I know I am trying to integrate the violence from my childhood. I can't do this with you. If you like it, I won't feel safe."

I was tearing up in spite of myself.

O's face softened. He nodded, visibly moved.

"Come here," he said.

I sat between his legs stretched out on the bed. Oz wrapped himself around me.

"Let's try. If it's too much we can stop."

We started watching, but after a few moments in I asked him again to stop the video.

"Tell me what's happening," O pleaded.

"I think she's being hurt…and I'm ashamed that it turns me on."

"Can I turn it back on?"

We did, and I was shaking. Oz watched the video, his head at a pensive tilt.

"It feels to me like she's acting. Look at her facial expression; she doesn't seem scared. They are playing at the dominant/submissive roles."

We watched it again several times, then put the computer away. Oz wrapped himself around me and started kissing my neck, then biting my nipples. I was wildly aroused. He took me with a confident forcefulness, and I felt undone—my feminist brain rewired.

After that night, Oz found interesting articles online and in the *New York Times* on women who viewed porn. He knew some of the porn and fantasies I was drawn to were attempts to integrate parts of my psyche that had encountered violence and emotional humiliation. We talked about my stepfather in this context, and Oz was exceptionally tender and supportive. It amazed me that a *man*—a classically *masculine man*—could witness my sexual split personality with intellect and compassion, and even help me through it. He also empathetically listened to my sorry-ass tales with an openness that inspired me to be even more vulnerable. It seemed to me that our roles had switched. Years ago, during our treasured walks, I had been the one to encourage him on a spiritual path of self-enlightenment. Now here he was, my loving travel companion on an unplanned journey to heal past trauma, integrate my authentic sexuality, and discover together how to hold feminism in this sexual exploration. We candidly discussed how our shadow sex play could be a vehicle to heal my splintered psyche, and Oz became my partner in doing so.

One morning after the kissing episode I came home with groceries to find Hank sitting on the couch. He had a sad look on his face. When I asked him what was up he said, "I am going through some stuff about us."

My throat tightened.

"What's up?" I asked.

"I feel grief about us. I know I signed off on this, but I feel so sad, like we're losing a part of us that we may never get back. It may be irrevocable what we're doing. You're usually the emotional one but..." his voice trailed off and he started to cry.

I sat down next to him. I was struck again by my lack of words. For so many years I had wanted him to need me. Now he needed me and it felt too late.

"I guess I felt that grief a long time ago," I said as I tentatively clasped his hand.

Hank was sitting back on the couch looking like a startled child. He nodded. I knew the impact of my words was huge. I felt an immediate compulsion to want to talk about what I saw as the next phase of our relationship. I wanted to keep going, to stay connected on this life journey. But I knew we could not be lovers again. We could be family—but not romantic. Too much time had passed for me in which potential erotic energy had laid dormant. But at this time, I was too scared to say I felt sexually done.

In my mind I was adding in a new person *and* still retaining my deep love and loyalty for Hank. I believed our relationship could continue but in a new form. I saw Hank and me as similar to my friend Lila and her husband, and other married couples I knew who were no longer having sex yet deeply bonded as family, aligned in raising their children, more like life mates than passionate lovers. In retrospect, this was perhaps presumptuous of me to want Hank to joyously accept this transition and adjust to huge changes in our relationship without a grieving period.

Hank was still a fundamental person in my life, and I hoped with all my heart that he would continue to be. He was just realizing the loss that was happening—the loss I had felt for years. But I was confident that although that night marked the end of us as romantic partners, it was also the beginning of a new phase in our relationship.

We estimated it would take roughly six weeks to prepare the duplex for Oz's kids to spend half their week with us. Oz asked his son how he would feel about living at Grace's house "sometime in the future." Liam became extremely excited about doing "sleepovers" with Merlin three times a week—both Merlin and Liam wanted more sleepovers. Tallulah had always wanted a little sister, so she was excited about bonding with Amy. Oz was elated that Liam felt comfortable with the idea. He prepared to talk with Susan.

The next day, Oz received an e-mail from Susan asking why Liam was saying he was moving in with Daddy at Grace's house. Oz explained that he was planning to give up his apartment and move in with me, and that he wanted to gauge Liam's reaction to the idea of living at Grace's house. Susan responded that it was unacceptable for her kids to live at my house. Oz reassured Susan that the household was a wonderful place, and he told her that the kids were already enjoying each other when they played here on the weekends. But she was not pleased.

Oz and Susan e-mailed back and forth all week. Oz read me some of the e-mails and we discussed how to respond. I suggested he be as transparent as possible, but nothing Oz said seemed to calm the situation down. I wondered if there was a way that we could all sit and talk, but things continued to escalate.

On Friday evening I met Oz after work in San Francisco. We walked to a hotel that had an infamous bar thirty-nine floors up. We sat in what felt like the clouds, drinking cosmopolitans. Oz had an exhausted, hollow look in his eyes. I tried to reassure him.

"Let's do what we need to do to avoid an ugly custody battle. It's not worth you getting emotionally and financially depleted."

Oz shook his head, "I lost it."

"What do you mean?"

Oz opened his phone and handed it to me. It was an e-mail he'd sent to Susan.

At no time have the children witnessed anything inappropriate nor will they ever witness anything inappropriate while under my care. I will not answer questions or give you details which do not relate to the kids' experience. As an example, you asked if I were having homosexual relations with Hank. I find such questions irrelevant and offensive to my right to privacy. There is a litany of such questions asked throughout history, which would best be answered with "None of your business." E.g. Sen. McCarthy asking, "Are you a communist, or associated with communists?" Hitler asking, "Are you a Jew? Are you a homosexual?" The Soviets asking "Are you practicing organized religion?" Even if the answer to any of these questions is no, I'd prefer to answer, "It's none of your business, I refuse to answer." For the record, the children have not experienced any drunken, sexual, orgiastic, hedonistic, communist, terrorist conduct while under my care.

I handed the phone back to Oz.

"Yikes."

Oz took a gulp of his drink. I was torn. As a parent I didn't want Oz to lose custody of his kids. I told Oz to put it in terms that she could understand: right now we weren't doing poly (which, by her definition, seemed to entail out-of-control sexual behavior in front of the kids). Currently we were two monogamous couples. We would be living on separate sides of the house, with locked doors and clear boundaries. I even suggested that Oz tell her Hank and I were separated so that it would fit into the societal map everyone felt comfortable with.

Later, Oz composed a long e-mail outlining exactly where people would be sleeping, and with whom. But when I read it, I proceeded to get completely depressed. Describing our living arrangement using divorce language did not capture the spirit of what we were doing. I told my friend Jocelyn about the e-mail. She tried to comfort me by saying, "But *you are separated*. You aren't having sex with Hank anymore. Isn't that one of the definitions of marriage—conjugal rights?" But I did not share this opinion. I still felt fully bonded and married to Hank. It was depressing to have to dumb it down and use language that didn't align with me.

Unwittingly, I had ventured into dangerous territory by allowing Susan to define us. I began to understand the perils of telling the interrogator what she wants to hear to make your life easier. I gained even greater respect for the actors and directors at McCarthy hearings who allowed their entire lives and careers to be ruined because they would not lie under oath just to get some peace. Once you have perjured yourself, you have lost the one thing that was carrying you through the whole mess: your sense of who you are, your belief in what is correct. I felt that the four of us should be able to live together under one roof loving each other and making a family with each other and our children. That this was seen as potentially perverse was disheartening.

How could I explain to Susan that it was unlikely that Hank and I would ever have sex again, but that I still considered him a husband and my family? I still loved him dearly. The truth of what we were doing was so much tamer than what she was probably imagining. At its simplest, we were just two couples living side by side, raising our kids, loving and respecting each other, and (me at least) in bed by nine p.m. Hell, we were boring. I didn't have the time, energy, or inclination for wild orgies.

The next day the doorbell rang and a man in a suit asked if Oz was available. I instantly knew what was going on. I said "No," then shut the door. I walked upstairs to get Oz.

"Babe, I think you are being served."

Just then Oz's cell rang. Oz stood holding his phone, and we stared at it like it was a hand grenade. Then the cell phone clanged, indicating a message had been left. Oz listened to it.

"Susan is taking me to court to prevent the kids from living here."

Oz walked downstairs and opened the door. He was served. The server thanked Oz for not making his job more difficult. We were in shock. What would we do if Oz's kids could not move in?

Chapter 16

I called my poly support group and got a referral for a lawyer who was poly and had defended poly cases. The day of the hearing, our lawyer was late. Oz and I sat like two nervous deer. Then she swept in and gave a speech to the judge about our parental rights and sexual freedom; her argument was that whether or not we were poly was inconsequential—we were still excellent parents.

Susan's deposition to the court stated that "the lifestyle choices of the three parents"—Hank, me, and Oz—"have taken precedence over the emotional needs of the children." And that Oz "addresses his own needs and completely ignores the needs of his children." Susan's lawyer stood and continued this absurd line of reasoning. She started to describe Oz. I was shocked. It was as if I'd walked into the wrong court hearing, one in which the father was a supreme creep—a horny deadbeat dad. Susan's lawyer was requesting a custody agreement whereby Oz would feed his kids dinner and put them to bed at Susan's house, or he would keep his apartment and live separately from me.

After our lawyers spoke, the judge asked, "Does the father have a separate apartment in which he can see the children?"

Our lawyer answered yes, and then the judge overruled our request to allow Oz's children to live half the week at my house and ordered a full evaluation by a court-appointed therapist. The evaluation would be an assessment of Oz, me, Hank, Valerie, and our home together. This also meant that Susan would be evaluated—but we were clearly the ones under scrutiny. The completed evaluation would ostensibly provide information for the judge to make a final ruling on where and with whom the children could live.

The judge told us that Oz's children could be at my house in the day but must sleep at Oz's apartment at night. This struck me as odd. If our home was actually a dangerous place for children, why allow the kids there at all?

We were assigned an evaluator. Our lawyer told us that the evaluator could show up at my house or Oz's apartment at any time unannounced and inspect the premises. *Huh. Would the evaluator also have a license to confiscate any sex toys or lingerie she found on site? Was she empowered to scold us for being sexually active parents and send us to bed with no dinner?* I was both amazed by and indignant about the proceedings. When we got back to my house Oz crawled into bed and stayed in the fetal position for half an hour. I sat next to him rubbing his back. He was terrified that he was going to lose his kids. I reassured him, but I was worried too. I prayed Oz would not be punished for our lifestyle.

It seemed we were not the only ones affected by the cloud of uncertainty shadowing us. One Saturday night at Oz's apartment we tucked Liam, Merlin, and Amy in their sleeping bags in the living room because they wanted to "camp out." Oz and I were snuggling in the bedroom when we heard a light knock on the door. Amy came in saying, "Daddy, I have a tummy ache."

Oz had confided in me that he felt a "tummy ache" was code for "needing more attention." Oz scooped her up in his arms and said with a warm smile, "Do you have a tummy ache or do you just need more love?" Amy looked confused, as if she didn't know the latter was an option. But it became clear pretty quickly that she just needed some of Daddy's attention. They sat out on the balcony, looking at the stars, Oz rocking her till she fell asleep.

Over the next few weeks our lawyer seemed scattered. Then one day she messed up a deposition that should have been sent to the judge. That night I had a dream with the clear message that if we did not get a new lawyer, we would lose the trial. I told Oz about the dream. He didn't want to make any big changes until after the evaluation. But the very next night I had a dream with even scarier images: us losing the trial and Oz's children never being allowed to live with us. I convinced Oz to let me find a new lawyer. He agreed.

The next morning I made a list of thirty lawyers who had been personally referred to me or whom I had found through my own research. After talking to three of them I was glad I had trusted my gut. It became clear that this was no time to sit back and relax. This was game time in terms of making a good impression for the evaluation. Even the lawyers who were clearly not right for us, the ones to whom I had to spell out my living situation like I was sounding out the alphabet to a toddler, warned me to get moving. They explained to me that the judge would pretty much be taking the evaluator's observations as conclusive evidence of what the children needed. We would be evaluated on everything pertinent to the children: *Were there handcuffs and leather whips mixed in with the LEGOS in the kids' toy box? Did I have a giant cauldron in our fireplace and deadly potions in an unlocked drawer labeled "candy"? A continuous feed of porn playing on my DVD? Should Susan get complete primary custody because we were so wrapped up in getting laid that the kids were playing croquet in oncoming traffic?* Whatever the evaluator concluded and recommended, the judge almost always adhered to.

As I interviewed lawyers and mediators, I described Hank and me living next to each other and continuing to parent our kids together. Several of them said, "That's a great situation for the kids." But they also told me that there had been no precedent-setting case for parental rights when a parent was poly. One lawyer told me being poly was uncharted territory in child-custody cases.

Toward the end of the day I spoke to an energetic lawyer whom I liked immediately. I explained how Hank and I were not having sex but still loved each other; we wanted our new partners, but also wanted to keep our family intact.

"You two sound like the poster children for co-parenting," she said. She started making recommendations on how to prepare for the evaluation. I hired her immediately.

I hoped that the judge would see us as the poster children of coparenting but I knew that we had quite a battle ahead of us to clear our reputation and explain what we were doing as parents. Our intention was that each member of our family (children and adults) would thrive. It seemed to me that family life requires a delicate balance of making sure you are well and happy and that your children are well and happy. Oz, Hank, Valerie, and I closely observed and responded to the needs of the kids. But the argument being put forth to the judge seemed to be that because we were actively pursuing sexual gratification we had no credibility as parents.

The accusation that Oz put his needs above his children's was not at all true to my experience of him as a dad. When Oz's kids were at my house on the weekends, he'd spend the entire day riding bikes around the block, playing hide-and-go-seek, reading to them. He did this not only with Liam and Amy but with Merlin and Tallulah as well. In fact, he focused so completely on the kids that he forgot basic things like doing the dishes or cleaning up. He was always onto the next thing that they wanted or needed. I thought all the playtime was great, and I would join in on the activities. But in no time my house would look like a bomb had exploded.

I was used to the workload of two kids, but soon my workload doubled. On Saturdays there were frequently four kids in my house. Of all the things to cause pain and conflict in our newfangled household, the last thing I anticipated were spats over chores. It seems housework is truly the great divider. At the end of all those Hollywood romances, if cinema aptly portrayed real life (which it does not, nor is it meant to) you would find the stars of the romance fighting bitterly over whose turn it was to do the damn dishes.

I felt that I was doing too many dishes. Valerie, unbeknownst to me, also felt she was doing too many dishes. When I heard this I was surprised. Hank wasn't your typical husband. He cooked, did laundry, and changed diapers. Our arrangement was generally fifty-fifty in the domestic-chores department. We didn't necessarily split each task, but we did split the amount of them. For instance, although I've never seen him scrub a toilet (I wasn't sure he even knew that toilets routinely had to be cleaned), I've enjoyed plenty of his home-cooked meals. While I mopped the kitchen floors, Hank vacuumed.

I asked Hank about Valerie and the dishes problem. What became clear was that Valerie was not accustomed to the staggering workload that kids created—dishes being just one fallout. Hank tried to explain to Valerie that although there wasn't symmetry in the chores he and I did, there was balance. However, it was becoming evident that the way we had balanced the chores wasn't working in the new living arrangement. Now that my kids were eating more often on Hank's side of the house, more work was piling up for Valerie and Hank. And I wasn't going to go over and scrub their kitchen after my kids ate there! My side of the duplex was turning out to be a funhouse for all four kids on the weekends. On top of that, my side encompassed the kids' bedrooms, so I was left with all the chores of tidying up two more rooms, an additional bathroom, and all of their laundry. I began to wonder if the great ideologies and manifestos throughout history were felled not by huge missteps but by simple, mundane failures—like no one putting their shoes in the damn closet.

I tried to woo the kids back onto my side of the house, but they complained about my cuisine. They'd peruse what I was making for dinner, then go over to Hank and Valerie's side. One time, after I had been sautéing a plate of vegetables for Merlin, he actually asked me, "Do you have anything that's less healthy?"

As if gastronomy issues weren't enough to daunt me, one day Oz presented me with yet another domestic enigma. He and I had set out to clean the kitchen. I was scrubbing each dish, then handing it to Oz to load into the dishwasher.

"Why are you washing the dishes?" he asked.

"Well, they won't get clean if I don't," I said.

"Your dishwasher is mechanically inferior."

"What?"

"Two words: Dish. Washer. If your dishwasher isn't *washing* your *dishes*, then what's the point?"

Even though my machine clearly sucked, I was a bit annoyed that Oz had the gall to say it out loud. He stated flatly that he was going to buy us a dishwasher, which he decreed would "decrease our workload and end our domestic quarrels." I was only half listening. I was sure this was a male-brain thing, like Hank and the self-scrubbing toilets. Oz just didn't get housecleaning.

But two weeks later, there was a glistening black machine in my kitchen. Oz suddenly got nervous as we loaded the dishes caked with dried food residue.

"I like to underpromise and overdeliver," he said. "Now I'm worried I've overpromised and the dishwasher will underdeliver. I hope this works."

I liked how earnestly he took the situation. Forty-five minutes later we opened the dishwasher and pulled out the tray. I picked up a shimmering, perfectly clean dish—and my life has never been the same since.

Oz immediately outlined a new domestic system: "A dish is either being used at the table or in the dishwasher." He coached the kids to clear the table and put their dishes directly into the dishwasher. And just like that our problems were—if not solved—immensely better. Who knew? I thought I had a sexism problem, when I really had a mechanical problem. I was delighted.

Word of the miraculous machine reached the other side of the house. Hank said to me, "I don't know if I should be insulted or happy that Oz replaced my dishwasher." Then Valerie asked if she and Hank could use it. How could I refuse? Soon we had to come up with elaborate schedules and dishwasher-sharing rules. But just as quickly, the sharing schedules got wacky. Hank and Valerie started sneaking their dishes in late at night, then boldly on a Saturday afternoon during prime time.

I told them I wasn't so keen on them using the dishwasher. After all, they both had been apathetic when I told them about my house-keeping woes: having the kids' bedrooms and bathroom and more square footage to clean on my side of the house. I explained that their extra dish loads were impeding my ability to keep my sink empty. We talked. We processed. For about eight weeks' worth of VHOGs, the dishwasher dominated discussions. Finally we all agreed it was best for Valerie and Hank to do their own dishes by hand on their side of the house, while researching the purchase of their own machine. I felt relieved to be done with the dishwasher episode—and also fascinated that it had caused such a stir.

It was Tallulah's birthday, and we were hosting a sleepover with five of her best pals. I was hustling to clean the house and download songs from *Glee* so that she and her friends could do *Glee* karaoke. Oz took Merlin, Liam, and Amy to a museum while Tallulah and I got ready to stock up on groceries. When I'd finished dressing for our foray to Berkeley Bowl, Tallulah started moaning like a little calf. I thought I looked *fine*, but she was mortified to be seen with me. I had just bought a fabulous dress, a sporty mauve sheath that I paired with leather boots and a vintage 1950s woolen cape, something Tippi Hedren might have worn in a Hitchcock film. I was excited to show it off at the grocery store. (Clearly I wasn't getting out enough).

While we walked through Berkeley Bowl Tallulah hissed, "Everyone is looking at you!"

"Isn't that the point?"

I was so excited people were looking at me. I hadn't bought any new clothes lately and my wardrobe was getting really dreary. It was pouring rain when we finished shopping, and I tied a silk scarf around my newly dyed red locks.

Tallulah keened, "No! You are embarrassing me!" through clenched teeth.

I compromised, asking her to hold the umbrella for me instead as I pushed the shopping cart and we darted back to the car.

Driving home, she had a complete meltdown about what her friends would think of our living arrangement.

"I want to be normal!" she wailed.

I sat in silence. After a few minutes she asked me what I thought.

I told her, "I empathize with you, and I know it is hard that no one else is doing it the way we are doing it. But I think it's great if people make choices that work for them. I am proud of us."

She shrugged, "I want us to be normal."

I felt torn. I wanted to give her normal, but I couldn't just fade into the background like bland wallpaper.

At home I cleaned, made cupcakes, and ordered the pizza. Oz helped set up the karaoke. He had become our Chief Technical Officer since moving in. Once, after Oz had hooked up all our computers, fixed the Wii when it crashed, trouble-shot our Internet connection, and got the printer running, he had said to me, "Baby, I am not the CTO. I am the OTO."

I asked, "What does that stand for?"

"I am the *Only* Technical Officer."

On Tallulah's birthday Oz spent two hours fixing the technical glitches with the microphones and downloading songs onto my laptop while the three younger kids played upstairs. At about four o'clock Tallulah pulled me aside.

"When is Oz leaving?" she asked.

Oh no, I thought.

We talked. She really wanted Oz to leave. She didn't know how to explain who he was to her friends. The odd thing was that she didn't feel the same way about Valerie. Valerie had been preparing a craft project—canvas purses to make with the girls—and she'd also made special snacks and popcorn for movie time. The double standard fascinated me. Valerie could be there with me, serving pizza and snacks, no questions asked. In other words, additional women were normal as long as they were serving you food.

Tallulah was very clear. Oz had to leave and leave *now*. The girls would be here soon. I tried to convince her to please let Oz stay. I pointed out that he'd been working all afternoon *to help her*. But she was almost panicked about him staying. So I went to Oz and tried to tell him the situation as delicately as I could, but it was rough. He got a wounded look on his face.

"We can't stay for pizza? Then I'll take my kids back to the apartment?"

I tried to explain that Tallulah was embarrassed. Oz went silent, and then he got morose. He asked Tallulah if he could just stay for some pizza. She started to cry. Then I wanted to crawl under the house and eat worms. It was just awful.

I finally said to Oz, "Please, this will get better. But can we humor her tonight?"

He left and took his kids out for pizza. An hour later I had to call him to get his telephone assistance through another technical glitch with the karaoke. He talked me through it for twenty minutes, after which I said, "Baby, you're a saint."

"No," he said, "I am just madly in love with you."

The morning after Tallulah's birthday, it was clear that I needed extra hands in the kitchen to make pancakes for all the girls. So I went through the door from my dining room into Hank and Valerie's kitchen. They weren't there. So I yelled for them up the spiral staircase. Valerie had asked me not to do it months ago. I had stopped for a while, but the house was so big and lumbering it was hard not to. If Hank wasn't in his kitchen, I had to hoof it all the way through my dining room and living room, up a flight of stairs, and knock on the hallway door that led into their living room. It was quite a workout!

That morning, I forgot about Valerie's request not to yell. A few minutes later I went back into their kitchen to get a broom. It was understood that it was okay to occasionally pop in and grab household items or a cup of sugar, if need be. That's when I overheard Valerie in their bedroom say, "I hate it when she does that!"

Then Hank replied, "So tell her."

"I did, and she is crossing my boundary."

I felt suddenly repugnant—an unwanted viral presence. Five minutes later Hank came to my kitchen. We talked as we made pancakes side by side. He said Valerie was not used to having so many people around and was stumped on how to set boundaries. Then Valerie walked in.

I said, "I heard what you said."

She replied, "Thanks for violating my boundaries!"

Then she walked out and we avoided each other all day. Then I got completely freaked out—I knew I was in the wrong and had to apologize, but I was frozen with fear that she might move out and take Hank with her. That night I lay in bed next to Oz. I was strobing through worst-case scenarios over and over again, my brain like a poly horror movie. Oz asked me what was going on, and I told him.

"Hmm," he said, propping his head up on his elbow. "When was the last fight you and Valerie had?"

"About six months ago."

"If you were to rate this interaction on a scale of one to ten, one being awful, ten great, where would it be?"

"A three."

"How often are you at a three with Valerie?"

"Rarely."

"What is the number you feel you are mostly at?"

"Things are usually great, so maybe we are consistently at an eight or nine."

"I'd say, if you put this on a graph, and did a time-averaged value, you'd be at an eight most of the time with a few glitches. Most likely, you'll be back at an eight soon."

I never knew a graph could calm me down so quickly. I felt immensely better, enough to fall asleep. The next day, Valerie and I made up. We had a good conversation. I apologized about calling up the stairs. She was gracious about the whole incident. We came up with ways that we could communicate better. Then we checked in about agreements in general.

Oz's counseling on the situation was a revelation for me. If I had sought advice from any of my artist friends we would have spent at least twenty minutes on what had been triggered from my child-hood, another twenty minutes describing in detail the situation and every person's viewpoint in the house, the neighborhood, and other parts of the world. We would probably have eventually reached the same conclusion that Oz reached in seconds, that this would all blow over quickly.

I was hoping that Oz's graph would apply to the court hearings. Although the evaluation was still hanging over us, we seemed to be trending toward smoother waters. Many of our friends had settled down and were supporting what we were doing. When I had dinner with my friend Jocelyn, she admitted that at first she'd thought what we were doing was "nuts." But her thinking had changed. Over the past year she'd decided to divorce her husband. She had discovered he'd been carrying on an affair for many years. Jocelyn had tried to salvage her marriage despite the revelation but couldn't get past the betrayal. When Hank and I had first started living a polyamorous life, Jocelyn had warned me to hire a lawyer; now she lauded our transparency and the integration of our new relationships. This had been the arc of most people upon hearing about our setup—alarmed at first but slowly calming down once they fully understood our intentions.

It had been hard to be a fish swimming upstream against the current of what was presently considered "normal" and "acceptable" in creating a family. I felt done caring about everyone's opinions about my iconoclastic life. All I cared about was whether our little family worked. *Are everyone's needs being met?* I was especially watchful of the children, who were sometimes unable to identify their needs, let alone express them. I'd even watch my little witch, now securely lodged in the awkward tween years, bask in the attention of us four adults—and wonder if things were working better for her. I wasn't quite sure how she was currently feeling about the addition of Oz and Valerie. Until one night, due to some bad restaurant food, I got my update.

"I'm going to throw up!" announced Tallulah from the couch, where she had been clutching her tummy for the past couple of hours.

I ran to get a bowl from the kitchen, when Tallulah vomited on the couch. Oz and I both rushed over to her. I helped her upstairs while Oz cleaned up, which was quite a shocker. Voluntarily cleaning up another's vomit ranks very high in my book of admirable character traits. I was helping Tallulah into the bathroom when Valerie came over to see if Tallulah was feeling better. As Tallulah leaned over the john, Valerie gave tips on how to manage the puking.

As I was settling Tallulah into bed, she said to me, "Oz is such a good person. And I love Valerie. Would you wake up Daddy?"

I knocked on Hank's door quietly. Throwing up was sacrosanct—you have to pay your respects. He came in and tucked Tallulah into bed.

When I came downstairs I said to Oz, "Tallulah had four adults loving her and helping her tonight. I can't help but feel we are doing it right."

"But not normal," Oz replied.

"Goddess forbid."

Even if Tallulah couldn't yet accept the unique family and home life I was determined to give her, I was certain her needs were being met.

My needs were finally being met behind locked doors, in the love den of my bedroom sequestered on a separate floor by itself. Because I had asked Oz to be exclusive and close our relationship for now, I was providing variety by playacting a plethora of women. I had become the Meryl Streep of sex play. Acting the role of a girl from college that Oz had an awkward make-out session with at a frat party then always regretted not dating; the bank teller with erect nipples who was extremely friendly every time Oz made a deposit; an exhausted waitress at his favorite vegetarian restaurant whom Oz felt sure he could invigorate with a love injection; pretty much any scenario was up for grabs, and it all turned me on too.

One night, after a marathon lovemaking session, Oz wistfully confessed to me another of his fantasies.

"I've always wanted to have anal sex."

"I did it once and came like a firecracker."

"Really?"

"Baby, you have a giant cock."

Oz was spooning me tightly from behind. I could feel his giant member brushing against my butt. I was excited by the idea but—

"I am not sure it's possible with you."

The perfect cock for anal was long and thin—definitely not Oz.

Then Oz said quietly, "You know, I'd be so scared to have anal sex with you. I've wanted it for so long. If I ever got it, I'd be so frightened that you'd go away but that I'd be hooked on you. Addicted forever."

Oz hooked on my ass throughout eternity—where do I sign up? At that moment I decided that, even if it killed me, I was going to get Oz's dick up my ass.

The next day bright and early I was at my computer researching the how-to of anal sex. I had fantasized about anal sex for years, and

I was excited to finally have an interested partner. But I was also scared, given all my ass had been through—I didn't want to literally reopen past wounds. I had always been intrigued by the root chakra, which assists us in feeling more grounded to the earth; with all the mental illness and instability of my caretakers, feeling solidly connected to people who sustained me had always been a challenge. *Instead of reopening old wounds, could I use anal sex to heal them?*

As I saw it, the highest sexual experience for me, both transformative and healing, would be to be sodomized by Oz. I imagined it would be the ultimate opportunity for sexual-spiritual unification. I was scared to open my ass and let Oz sexually dominate me, and probably because of my fear it was also a tremendous turn-on that my Romeo was enthused to enter my dark recess.

A few days later, I tracked down *the* book on anal sex for women by a sexpert on the topic. It was an impressive guide, outlining how to work up to anal penetration. Apparently a woman had to be extremely turned on, sloppy wet, and ready—to easily take a cock up her ass. There was a quote from a guy who said, "I don't even get near my lady's ass until I've given her a few clitoral orgasms." *I liked the philosophy.* I read the section to Oz, who had the typical male fantasy that he'd just flip me over and pummel away porno style.

Oz told me he had been chatting with an ex-girlfriend when he told her of our plans. She snorted, "If Grace takes your cock up her ass, she'll be my personal hero." It was a bit daunting to find that another gal in the Oz Girlfriend Club had deemed it an impossible feat.

I started playing with the dildo (we'd nicknamed it "The Rectal Engineer") on nights when Oz was at his apartment, earnestly trying to get the damn thing up my ass. I thought I'd be more able to open myself masturbating. No such luck. When we were together, Oz would stare with longing at my puckered rosebud—making me feel both fragile and adored. The book by the sexpert cautioned that anal sex should never hurt, and don't expect to get there in one night. So between the attacks on our character in court and attempted penetration by Oz's super-sized cock, my ass remained a no-entry zone.

I didn't feel defeated, though. In fact, every day I acknowledged with gratitude that I was beginning to achieve what I had wondered if was even possible a year ago. *Could I be a devoted mother and, at the same time, a lusty woman getting her carnal needs met too?* Although it could possibly fly in the face of the stony judgments of the evaluation, the answer was, apparently, yes.

Chapter 17

I was beginning to have the community I'd always longed for. Valerie had been officially moved in for several months. Although Oz still had his apartment, where he was required to sleep with his kids three nights a week, having him the other four nights felt amazing. Going from chance, forbidden encounters at the elementary school, to dating, to getting Oz four nights a week—and still having Hank—felt miraculous. Even though Oz's kids still could not sleep over, we were bonding as a family and I was thrilled. I'd always wanted a big family.

In the evenings when I opened up a bottle of wine, I'd frequently bring a glass over to Valerie. I liked chatting with her and listening to her thoughts and observations on the kids. Every day when I woke up and took my shower, I would stand under the hot water and muse over my life. *I was living with Oz and Hank and my kids. I had it all. How did I pull this off?* My brain would reel at the wonder of it.

We were living the dream but under siege. Susan and her lawyers were very busy. A deluge of court depositions written for the evaluator were being cc'd to us by Oz's lawyer. Oz felt he had become the poly whipping boy. He was shocked by the vitriol and reluctant to respond. His impulse was to ignore the attacks.

Oz had wanted an amicable divorce. He had aspired to have a peaceful closure and ending of his marriage to Susan with a new focus on co-parenting their kids. Oz wanted what Hank and I had: to be close and respectful, possibly even friends. But this was clearly not going to happen.

When the court hearings started, I said to Judy, my therapist, "I feel like I am being attacked."

She replied, "That's because you *are* being attacked."

It was difficult reading about myself in the court declarations. At times I would feel disbelief. Other times as if assaulted by artillery. As the case against us heated up, I melted down. I meditated more often and strived to distance myself from the personal nature of the accusations. I was written about in the court documents peripherally, in what I considered a scandalous tone. One line grated on me immensely. Susan's lawyer quoted Liam as saying, "Grace doesn't read to her kids." This was laughable and incorrect, and it was searing to my very core—my reputation as a mother being burned at the stake.

The case against us was simple in its uniformity. We were poly, therefore we were bad parents. It was such a straightforward trajectory that it had me wondering if I were missing something.

Was it bad to be a devoted parent who also prioritized getting laid? To me our living situation seemed like a great solution to our problems. My kids had access to their mother and father whenever they wanted them. I got to have my new lover and keep my family intact. And I was extremely open to sharing my house with Oz's kids as well.

Susan was demanding that Hank and I live on different premises if Liam and Amy moved in. She stated in court documents that she did not want her children part of a household that allowed for Hank to be close by. Interestingly, this would have forced the typical two-household divorce scenario for my children as well. How that could be viewed as more wholesome for our kids was beyond me.

If the judge decided we couldn't have Oz's kids live with us, we'd never have the opportunity to be a family together. It would mean a lifestyle in which Oz and I would only be together a few nights a week. I just couldn't understand why my being close to Hank was weird to everyone. It was almost as if people could not fathom Hank and I still loving each other. At the time, Oz used to scratch his head saying, "I just don't get it. Everyone would be so much more comfortable if you and Hank hated each other. Isn't that crazy?" It *was crazy*.

Where was the middle ground? A way for spouses to transition to a different place, satisfying everyone's needs and still remaining family—why was this so unheard of and threatening?

Around this time, I got a glimpse of how others might be seeing me. I attended a PTA fundraiser where one of the mothers started talking about her neighbor, a woman who had recently remarried and had two teenage boys. The mother said her own adolescent son slept over at this neighbor woman's house. Apparently her son went to get a soda from the fridge after midnight and heard the newly married couple having sex. I was about to say something like, "Oh, good for her!" when this mother said with disgust, "Can you believe her children are being exposed to that?"

At times like these I felt that if I spoke up I would likely get stoned. Oz and I were careful to lock the door before sex, and our bedroom was sequestered on a different floor from the kids, but I silently wondered if you were supposed to stop having sex after marriage rather than risk that your kids might—Goddess forbid—hear a few moans coming from your side of the house late one night. Was this really superior parenting? After that one night when you conceived your child, was all other sexual contact lascivious and antifamily?

One afternoon when the kids were at school, Oz and I spontaneously started making love. I had graduated from bank tellers and missed love to strippers—which I found infinitely more satisfying, fashion-wise. Oz was no longer asking permission to go to strip clubs because I was serving it up at home, dressed in the tackiest stripper's heels I could order online.

I was still devoted to the ass project, but it was proving to be more challenging than I anticipated. At first I'd felt like I had when I taught myself to blow-dry my hair from YouTube how-to-videos: *I am a resourceful, intelligent girl. How hard could this be?* I mean really thousands—maybe millions—of women were taking massive cocks up their asses in porn videos on a daily basis. *I can do this.*

But I was beginning to think it might not happen. Oz's cock was just too big, and *the motherfucker hurt*. For a few weeks we had explored with slender dildos and his fingers. Oz would put a second finger up my ass when he was behind me doggy style. It was a wild turn on. Then he'd move to put the tip of his dick in, and I'd try to relax, but panic would tighten my sphincter and Oz would immediately back off.

On this day, Oz had warmed me up appropriately while I lap danced for him for a good thirty minutes. That's when he offered me another "hundred bucks" if I'd "take it up the ass." With panache, I guided him into position. I felt ready, like this might be the moment at long last.

Just then his cell phone jingled with Susan's special ring. Oz reluctantly disengaged, fearing it might be an emergency with his children. But Susan was calling to inquire why Oz kept packing pepperoni in Liam's lunch when he wasn't eating it. The image of him, nude, holding his massive cock in his hands, while he sincerely tried to attend to the parenting matter at hand will remain indelibly etched in my mind.

I felt solidly that we were excellent parents, and being sexual did not change that, though I did sometimes wonder with anxiety what my community was thinking of my situation. I frequently ran an internal courtroom drama in my brain, justifying my position. I had an inner monologue explaining every nuance of our lifestyle, but in real life it was hard to talk directly to people about what we were doing.

There wasn't language to accurately describe it. Once, I told a Pilates client who was curious what was going on that Hank and I had "separated." She immediately got a pained expression on her face and said to me, "I am so sorry!" This felt completely wrong to me. I felt triumph not sorrow. At the next VHOG we discussed what I could say to clients if they asked. Hank said he didn't like me using the word "separation" to describe our situation. It was "the language of divorce." Valerie chimed in, "All divorce language is about sub-traction, and we are adding people in without subtracting anyone."

We decided that even if it made for less-concise conversation, we would not dumb it down. If someone asked, we could say, "We have evolved our relationship to..." It was cumbersome but worth it. Sometimes I'd bump into people from the neighborhood at the library with my kids or on the sidewalk in front of our house as I unloaded groceries. One neighbor said to me, "I see you! I see Hank! But I don't see you and Hank together...?" He had obviously seen Oz, the worst offender of public displays of affection, grab and kiss me on the sidewalk.

I was in a rush so I just smiled and said, "We're very together!" If a person was a friend or someone I wanted to draw closer, I'd spend the extra five minutes to outline what we were doing. The others had to stay in confusion. One brash neighbor asked me (again on the sidewalk in front of our house), "Are you doing poly?" I appreciated her straightforwardness. But I felt reluctant to give everyone a break-down of who was sleeping with whom. And that was what people seemed to want to know. The elevator speech I concocted was, "We are doing emotional poly. Our relationships are currently closed, but we do embrace a poly philosophy. I love Hank very much, but we aren't romantic anymore." But this became a long speech and one that I didn't know was true; who knew what Valerie and Hank's current agreement was?

Helping my neighbors understand what we were doing was the easier of the tasks at hand. Hank was struggling in this new stage of our relationship. One night Hank and I went out for a drink. We went to a bar that had Dark and Stormys on the cocktail menu.

I commented, "That's Oz's favorite drink, a Dark and Stormy."

"What do I care what Oz's favorite drink is? I don't give a shit."

I was stunned and went to the bathroom to make a mayday call to Reenie.

She told me, "He's hurt. Just try and hang in with him."

It seemed like sound advice, but I was unnerved by his anger.

A few weeks later I got another jolt. Tallulah had asked us to sit shivah for our cat, Tulip, who had died a few days before. I mixed some martinis (with kosher olives in honor of the occasion) for Hank and me. We were mildly tipsy and in an odd, vulnerable state, mourning for our family cat. Conversation strayed, and I don't know what crazed bee got stuck in my bonnet, but I asked Hank, "Hey, how often do you and Valerie have sex?"

"Oh, let's not talk about that."

The bee in my bonnet was buzzing. "Just tell me; you can tell me."

"Let's not discuss it."

I don't know what I was trying to accomplish. But I pressed on and finally Hank said, "Every time we're together."

My happy busy bee was crushed by the fly swatter of life. I immediately withdrew into a cocoon of depression. Hank touched my hand and kind of clasped it. He made a comforting cooing sound.

"That's it? That's all you got?" I said.

I was stunned and hurt by what I perceived as his meanness. It was obvious to me he was trying to wound me. So I had blown it by asking him about sex—which had always been a sensitive area in our relationship. But was it necessary to send a salvo missile back?

He looked sorry but also a little pleased with himself. I got up and left the room. An hour later I heard Oz's key in the door as I lay curled up in the fetal position in bed. Oz had never seen me this vulnerable. I knew he would try to comfort me. But I just wanted to lie there in my blood and puke till morning, when I could call Reenie on the East Coast. When he saw the look in my eyes, Oz made a gallant effort to bring me back from the dark side. He had a contin-ued fascination with my relationship with Hank. When he heard what had happened, he agreed that Hank was hurting and out for revenge. Oz felt empathy where Hank was concerned. After the light box exhibition, when I told Oz I wasn't really interested in having sex with Hank again, Oz had said, "I hope you never feel that way about me."

That night Oz tried to convince me that I was the most gorgeous and desirable woman in the Universe, which only made me more depressed. I told him I'd feel better after I talked with a best friend and neutral observer. The next day Reenie and I dissected the situation.

I said, "I can't quite put my finger on it but it's something like that whole idea of my love not being good enough to crack him open. What does Valerie have that I don't have? It's worse than thinking you may be physically unattractive; it's the knowledge that Hank knows me more intimately than practically anyone and yet has rejected me sexually."

"I think our boy Hank is having some pain about the new arrangement."

"But he's getting laid every time they're together!"

"Yes, that may be true, but flip the tables. What if Hank came to you and asked you about your sex life with Oz. What would you say?"

I thought about it for a second. "I'd completely play it down; I wouldn't give any specific details. I'd focus on making him feel loved."

"Exactly," Reenie said.

As the Universe would have it, the day after this colossal punch in the stomach Hank and I had to embark on a previously planned trip to Los Angeles to visit his mom and dad. We would have six hours in the car side by side when I was barely talking to him.

When we got into the car to go pick up the kids at school, Hank asked, "Can we talk?"

"I'm not sure. I don't want to be hurt anymore."

"Look, I'm really sorry. I crossed a boundary with myself. I don't want to know about you and Oz sexually, and I promised myself that if you ever asked I wouldn't tell you anything. I'm sorry."

"Okay, I accept your apology."

"Is there anything you want to process before we get the kids?"

"Like what?"

Hank laughed, "Gee, there's not much going on in our lives, huh?"

But after several hours in the car things had morphed. We were doing a personality test from a book I got at the library. I read him the list of five creative styles. We picked one describing him. Then we both pondered me. He picked "c" but was still mulling it over. I read it again: "You are c) highly creative, self-absorbed, and moody."

"Gosh, I am really stuck on this one," Hank said, "because I don't see you as moody."

I couldn't stop laughing. There was something about someone knowing me for so long and telling me I was self-absorbed, but still worth it, that made it better. It wasn't that I even agreed that I was self-absorbed. I was absorbed with healing, which I guess could get tedious to listen to. For so many years I had idealized Hank. I literally could not see one thing that was wrong with him. I remember a brief moment of buyer's remorse after our wedding when he kept endlessly adjusting the sheets like a cat claws its bed before sleeping in it.

But now I could see his flaws, as he could mine—but he was still lovable. I had no desire to go through a laundry list of blaming each other for mistakes made in the past twenty-five years together. I was in a place of gratitude of what we had created together—our children, our healing, and the love we made together. I have always been a person who takes responsibility for making myself happy. I hoped Hank would do the same for himself and let me continue to be a part of his world—flaws and all.

Suddenly I felt like a member of a club I had never had the qualifications to be admitted to. Over the years, I'd listen with horror at people's descriptions of their family holiday dinners so dreadful that they made me feel relieved that my parents were dead. But then they'd describe the chicken soup that arrived when they were sick or the hike in the woods after the holiday carnage. These people had "good-enough family." I was beginning to understand what that meant.

Over the next few months Hank snapped at me a few times. I surprised myself by remaining calm. I felt like a cheerleader for a new kind of loving, but a cheerleader who was getting smacked around a bit by the other players and booed off the field. Under normal circumstances I could be a bit of a pit bull, biting the ankle of the offender as quickly as you could mumble "immature retaliation." But I tolerated Hank's occasional barbs, setting limits without poking back.

My tolerance was motivated by a bit of fear—possibly from ingrained family patterns whereby I put up with too much. But the other piece was that Hank was "good-enough family." He was my chosen family, and I felt a deep loyalty. After much contemplation on the subject, I kept coming up with the same answer. It was appropriate to be loyal with Hank. He was worth it. Hank had stood by me at a time when I had had no one else in the world. My loyalty felt emotionally correct. I didn't have enough family. Hank was my family.

Hank's presence was immensely soothing to my nerves. I liked his DNA. I was not one of those women who had always wanted kids; it was after being with Hank for more than a decade that I came to a place where I wanted babies—but only with Hank. I loved who he was and expected him to be a great father. I was not disappointed.

Sometimes I missed it just being me and Hank and our two kids. My nerves could barely handle the volume, the noise, the sprawl of *four* kids who were usually on my side of the house. The culture of Oz's family and his DNA were so different from the family culture Hank and I had created. Valerie had a similar vibration to Hank and me. She was arty, curious, and observational. Sometimes when I was overwhelmed on my side of the house, I'd knock timidly on Valerie and Hank's door. Tallulah would be already in their living room, sipping tea on the couch. They'd all be laughing and talking quietly. I'd moan from the threshold, "Could I come in for a bit?" I dubbed their side of the house "Sweden" and would occasionally ask for asylum.

I'd walk in and it would be like I was moving from the set of a loud superhero action movie to a French foreign film, with soft music playing in the background. The coffee table covered with take-out Indian food, candles flickering, the quiet timbre of Hank's voice—it all soothed me. I liked both sides of the house, and both sides of my life.

There were moments when I felt the bounty of having a big family and it thrilled me. When it worked, it really worked. For instance, one day I took Liam and Merlin for ice cream. We bumped into one of Liam's friends at the ice cream shop. Liam hooked his arm around Merlin's shoulder and proudly said, "This is my brother." Merlin looked down shyly and kicked the floor.

Somehow I thought we'd get to skip the stepparent issues, but we were clearly in the blended family tabloid (with a poly twist). At first Oz was just another big playmate for Merlin, but then he started to get hip to the fact that Oz was Mommy's boyfriend—and this did not sit well.

Merlin went through a period when every time I hugged Oz he'd whine, "Why do you hug Oz and you never hug Daddy?" I explained to him that I loved Daddy and that Oz was my new partner. He was inconsolable, wanting me to "kiss Daddy." One day Hank was passing through our kitchen when Merlin was playing Wii with

Liam. I grabbed Hank and said "Merlin, look!" then I planted a kiss on Hank. Merlin shrugged. There was no pleasing these kids.

Tallulah continued to be a kid who could predict what was coming up in the next six months, while I was still trying to paint a happy face on it. I didn't want to think or talk about my relationship with Hank in divorce language. But there was no denying that we were no longer husband and wife in the traditional scenario. It was exhausting not to have others on the block, down the street, or in the media who I could point to and say, "We are like the Jones family! See how they are still best friends, ten years after they moved their partners in?" I did have pals in the poly community, but everyone's experience was so vastly different that there were no clear parallels.

Sometimes I just felt exhausted by trying to help my kids through all the changes. I wanted to shout, *What do you kids want from my life?! I clean, worry, scrub, cook, listen, help with homework, put a roof over your head, wake up at five a.m. to see clients to buy you food, clothes, and useless toys that I see strewn on the floor within twelve hours of purchase. Now you think you can dictate who I get it on with? Who thought of this screwy system? It is completely insane to put children in charge of your well-being.*

But we did seem to be in a new workable stage in terms of creating a family together. Around this time I was dubbed "Gracie." It started with Amy. One, day, in her clear little voice, she had called "Gracie!" from the living room as I made her favorite pesto noodles in the kitchen. Tallulah and Merlin latched on to my new handle—but I put a stop to that tout de suite.

"It's 'Mom' to you," I said to my little babes. I hadn't gotten fat and gone through hard labor for a first-name-casual relationship. I wanted the high grade M-O-M status. But with Amy, Liam, and the adults, oddly enough, Gracie stuck. Even Oz started whispering it to me late at night; from his husky voice "Gracie" sounded like a burlesque queen. When I was a kid, both Reenie and my grandmother had used the pet name. Now, Amy's revival of my childhood nickname felt like a rebirth. An old part of myself was suddenly new again in my ever-evolving life. I imagined Gracie: a jaunty, bold gal, love connoisseur, relationship renegade!

Aside from my new moniker, another thing that kept me going was the love of Oz. The passion and urgency of our sex life did not decline. This amazed me and I wanted to know why it was working—so I could keep it working. When I shut the door at night in our love nest downstairs, it was as if the angels sang. I felt like Snow White after she'd ditched the queen with the poison apples, and birds sang and landed on my extended fingers. Rainbows popped out of the clouds, orgasms abounded.

One night Oz was inside me, pumping away. Another girl might have found him a bit rough, but I loved how his huge cock banged against my cervix like a farm boy clanging the dinner bell. In the midst of this rigorous pounding, at my request, Oz described last year's summer visit to a strip club. We had discussed our agreements at length before he went.

When deciding on the parameters, I asked, "Do strippers give blow jobs?"

He had answered like a shocked pontiff, "Goodness, no!"

So I had imagined some antiseptic booty dance, with said stripper at arm's length giving him a visual treat. At the time, Oz was truly stressed with his divorce and angst over not being able to live with me. He said he needed a "vent" to relieve his mounting anxiety. The strip club visit seemed like a necessary concession in a situation that was in gridlock.

As Oz plunged into me, the details of his visit were a wild turn-on: the woman he chose, walking her back to the booth, removing her clothes, biting her nipples, her riding his cock (albeit snugly tucked in his jeans). I came so forcefully I had to catch my breath. But once my breath had been caught I clawed a trail of skin off Oz's back. Oz howled in pain. The emotional whiplash from turn-on to indignation startled us both. Oz grabbed my hands and pinned them to the bed. I was laughing but also sincerely pissed off. *That was no antiseptic booty dance! That was sex!*

Thus began several hours of tense discussion as to what constituted sex, which I had not agreed to. Oz took the Bill Clinton line: no penetration, no sex. I told him in that case, could I spend an afternoon with a close friend rubbing his cock back and forth over my nether lips—since it wasn't sex? This caused Oz to groan loudly with frustration. For days we debated and discussed. I cooled down. We talked. We talked some more. The path we had chosen was a path of verbosity. We finally agreed that Oz had been remiss in describing what a lap dance entailed, which was unfair. He had raised a lot more sexual energy with the stripper than I was expecting.

We explored raising sexual energy with other people. We discussed again what we wanted around "openness." We were still getting used to having each other, and we felt protective of our relationship. One of my friends who went to play parties with her husband said that making love postparty was amazing, even if they just watched during the party. Oz's trip to the strip club seemed to have the same effect on us. It became endless fodder for our sex life. When Oz was inside me, with much coaxing—the boy had rightly become wary—he told me about all nine trips that he'd taken to strip clubs. They might as well have been nine million trips for all the psychic weight they held for me, but the descriptions of each trip made for an incredible erotic ride. Part of me saw Oz's sexuality as a feminist affront—it was feral and untamable. But this affront was a wild turn-on. When Oz went on business trips I would masturbate over him—which astonished me. Playing in this fantasy world— having a lover whose sexuality felt dangerous, but whose entire presence in my love was safe and regenerative—was healing. It was the sexual shadow play I had dreamed of having.

Our negotiations around openness in our relationship, though threatening at times, charged things up between us. I wasn't interested in hiring a sex worker, but it did appeal to me to possibly meet up with a woman from OkCupid. This felt too threatening to Oz, who was worried that I would become emotionally attached. It was conceivable that we'd never make it to a play party or have "golden tickets" (a limited pass to be sexual with other people). But the idea that this was a possibility, that we were still separate sexual beings with infinite amounts of mystery yet to be discovered, was a relationship plateau I could see riding for years.

One evening, I was mooching food over on Hank's side of the house. Frankly, I missed his cooking. Oz was a bit of a haphazard cook, and on the nights he was in charge of dinner, I had to babysit him with texts: "Have you put on the rice?"

Oz was at his apartment and Valerie was off in San Francisco, so it was just me and the kids with Hank. Hank stood slicing sausages and some parsley to go into a pasta primavera. I had brought my own wine to offset my mooching. After eating, Hank and I started talking about our first real estate project in San Francisco nearly twenty years ago, the earthquake shack we renovated while living in it.

Hank had hired a handyman in his early twenties to help finish the renovation. He had come cheap, and we had to constantly refocus him. I'd be typing out a play, Hank would be hammering, and our handyman would start a reverie about the latest headbanging concert he'd been to. We'd have to stop, redirect him, and say, "Work, hammer, build."

I started laughing so hard I had to put down my wine. Tallulah climbed into my lap like a lean cat and snuggled against my chest.

"I love it when you and Daddy laugh together," she said.

My eyes found Merlin. He was watching the scene with a hesitant smile on his face.

He said quietly, "You and Daddy really love each other."

"Yes," I said, "I love Daddy."

His little being glowed as I took him off to get his evening bath and nighttime story. I genuinely loved Hank and did not have to fake that. I celebrated the fact that I had procreated with him, and that was the essence of what my kids seemed to need, the knowledge that I loved both pieces of their DNA and that they were in a stable place. The performance kisses didn't do much. But the awareness that we were still part of a home where people love each other—that was the real thing.

Chapter 18

It was April. We'd been going through the evaluation for more than four months—and almost nothing was happening. The evaluator was moving at a snail's pace. We were in legal purgatory, paying tremendous legal fees with no end in sight. Oz was going crazy living in two locations: my house and his apartment. On Thursday, Friday, and Saturday, Oz had to sleep at his apartment because he had his kids. Although his apartment was only about ten minutes away from my home, it was wreaking havoc on his life. During the past several months, his cell phone would frequently die because the charger was always at his "other home." Food was constantly spoiling at his apartment as a result of his buying too much and then being at my home half the week. His apartment was always a mess because as soon as the kids went back to Susan's house Sunday morning, I'd start whining for his return.

One day Oz said to me, "Let's never buy a second home."

Amid all the shuffle, we were constantly on the defensive against potential scrutiny. But I refused to believe we'd lose. It just could not happen. How could anyone possibly look at what we were doing and not admire our commitment to our children and each other? But this vantage point alone made me nervous because I have always been someone who was out of touch with mainstream thinking. My gay friends had to explain step by step what homophobia was all about. I just couldn't get past "What do they care if I love a girl or a boy? Why would they want to rain on my parade?" I didn't read the papers or listen to the news. We were at the mercy of mainstream culture, and there was so much crazy injustice in the world that if I contemplated it, I'd break out in hives.

Oz had had two meetings with Edna, the court-appointed evaluator, whom we dubbed Edna the Evaluator. Oz was very suspicious of her; she'd rain on us for sure. But I was fully confident that once she met me and our family and saw what a nice girl I was, she'd write an evaluation that was like a love letter. I wanted to invite the evaluator to move in for a week. *We are fantastic parents—come see for yourself!*

I was proud of the way we navigated complex situations. For example, as we approached our first Mother's Day I felt some grief that there was another mother figure around. It seemed that one of the big payoffs for all the effort and toil you do as a mother was that no one could upstage you. You had the holy grail of parenthood; you were *The Mother.* No matter how wacky or grumpy you got, you were the birth canal, the boob, the vessel to life; you were the star of the household show wrapped in cellulite and fatigue.

Valerie was so peppy—taking the kids on special little outings after I'd spent the morning haranguing them to clean their rooms. She had the fun supporting role that historically stole the show from the star. The week before Mother's Day there was a pagan arts and crafts fair that Tallulah, Merlin, and I usually attended. The morning of the fair I went to get Tallulah. She told me she was going shopping with Valerie. I tried to cajole her to attend the fair, but she refused.

A couple of hours later, Merlin and I returned with ceramic Pan horns, candy apples, a beaded belt, and a saber. I had lavished him with gifts thinking for sure Tallulah would regret her decision. But she gazed at Merlin's horns and said, "Valerie has a friend who makes those. I'll just get a pair from her."

My shopping revenge foiled, I collapsed internally and went to pour myself a hefty glass of Chardonnay. Tallulah followed me downstairs.

"What's wrong?" she asked.

But I was mute with jealously and ashamed—my soul had shriveled.

Tallulah persisted, "Mommy, what's going on?"

I rallied my forces so she wouldn't feel guilty. We knocked on Hank and Valerie's door; they were snuggling on the couch. I asked if we could have "an emergency family meeting."

"Sure," Hank said.

"Next week is Mother's Day and I am struggling with having another mother figure in the house."

"I admire how honest you are in these situations," said Valerie.

I sat down. We all contemplated my opener.

Then Valerie offered, "I feel jealous when the four of you are together."

Just last week, after some negotiations, Valerie agreed to let just Tallulah, Merlin, me, and Hank have an outing together.

"Mommy, I'm sorry!" Tallulah said.

"Honey, you didn't do anything wrong. I want you to be close to Valerie."

"I don't ever feel jealous," said Tallulah.

"How would you feel if I took Amy to get a pedicure?" I asked.

Tallulah's face got stony. "No way!" she said.

Hank added. "I sometimes get jealous when Merlin wants to go play with Oz on your side of the house."

Once we had voiced our jealousies, we all calmed down. I loved the idea of sharing people. If I worked on my fears, I could allow a space for my kids to get more love. Valerie's presence was upping my parenting game. When she took Merlin and Tallulah to do a "smell walk" collecting aromatic plants, I asked myself, *What fun excursions have I done with them lately?* It inspired me to spend more quality time with them.

But that Mother's Day turned out to be challenging in an unexpected way. Hank, Valerie, Oz, and I went to a park with Tallulah and Merlin. We threw around a football and ate a picnic lunch. Several friends showed up and we toasted the moms. That evening, Hank and I had a moment alone on his side of the house. He gave me a pair of workout pants that fit me perfectly. The card read, "To my lovely wife." I felt self-conscious. Hank had never been one to emphasize terms like "wife."

"I wanted to ask you if, in the future, we could rekindle our sex life? I still think you're a beautiful woman and would love to have that connection."

I sifted through my brain to find the right words.

In the empty pause, Hank said, "I can see by your face that that isn't what you want."

"I guess I am not feeling that way anymore."

There was a stretch of silence. I suddenly yearned for the kids to burst into the room and interrupt us. When they didn't, I decided to delve into something I'd been curious about for a while.

"I'm wondering…over the years we had less and less sex. Weren't you ever concerned about not putting energy into *us*? What did you think was going to happen?" I asked it as gently as possible. I wasn't angry, although I had been angry in the past.

"I figured things would eventually turn back around again."

I nodded. I thought about the life of our relationship. I frequently had anxiety that Hank would leave (partially due to the chaos in my childhood), so I had a natural inclination to continually check in with him. If something wasn't working, I tried to change it. When Hank needed time for himself after we had kids, I encouraged him to take a weekly boys' night out.

But in Hank's culture, divorce was rare, and all his parents' friends stayed married for fifty years—till death do they part. But there were jokes about some of these couples and their constant bickering—even dislike of each other. In Hank's world, there was the "we'll never separate" assumption. But had that killed the eroticism and the emotional responsiveness in our relationship? Did Hank's "till death do us part" make him lackadaisical about my needs and responding to them?

Once, we were a playing a board game with several couples. A question was asked: "What is the biggest mistake you've made in the last five years?" People said things like "taking that job at the start-up," "not making it to my mother's deathbed." Hank sat stumped for several minutes, then his eyes gleamed and he scribbled an answer. When it came his turn, he read, "Not picking out the right movie at the video store." For years, I teased Hank about having the highest self-esteem I'd ever met in anyone. But I've come to the conclusion that it wasn't really about having high self-esteem. Did his certainty about his perceptions put him in a place where he rarely unpacked what was not working?

For years, I had talked to Hank about places in our relationship (mainly sex and money) that were not working for me, but he was able to turn down the volume of my requests. He was in a "till death do us part," nonurgent place, in a "we'd get there eventually" frame of mind. But I needed someone more like myself, hunting for any place that my partner felt unfulfilled and responding to those needs with urgency. One thing was for sure, I would never allow myself to be the identified wacko again. I trusted my emotional intelligence and vowed that it would be my compass in a relationship.

The court battle became so toxic that I began to find myself irritated by the enormous amounts of energy it took to deal with the attack. I was sickened by the expensive lawyers and the things being written about Oz. I was also genuinely baffled by how, after so many years of marriage, their connection had become so brittle, with no resiliency at all, even when it came to figuring out what was best for the kids. Where was the ability to maintain some love?

Oz felt empathy for Susan and wanted to take care of her. He believed it was possible to bring the poly philosophy into his failing marriage by continuing a loving connection. Oz would say, "We've been taking care of each other for ten years; there's got to be a way I can still take care of her." But when the court battle began and Oz read the depositions that repeatedly blasted his parenting, he gave up. He said to me, "Just last year Susan went on a vacation with her sister and didn't worry about me watching our kids. She thought I was a good dad back then."

Oz felt he was getting punished for wanting to live differently. And it did seem that he was being maligned for choosing to leave. The fact that he had spent years in therapy trying to create a different marriage was barely acknowledged in the court documents. But I could also understand Susan's viewpoint. She had signed up for a certain kind of relationship and Oz had completely changed the orientation of his life. What I could not understand was the attack. I understood the hurt, the grief, even the anger. But where was the compassion for how much effort Oz had invested in trying to create a marriage that worked for both of them?

Around this time, a longtime friend told me a story of watching a news show with her husband. It was on depression medication. On the show it said that one out of every four Americans is currently on Prozac. Her husband turned to her in disbelief, "That's astonishing. I don't know anyone on Prozac. Do you know anyone on Prozac?"

"You idiot," she said, "*I am on Prozac.*"

When she told me we laughed. But it got me thinking about how some marriages seemed to consist of two parallel lives. Like two trains side by side chugging down tracks, with the same destination—retirement, accumulated wealth, grown children, death. But this existence could just as easily be that of strangers occupying separate emotional—possibly sexual—worlds. In this scenario I could understand the sudden implosion of a marriage. If one person jumped off the tracks and the other wanted to keep chugging along, the marriage could get ugly suddenly.

I felt so differently about Hank. Our love had so many dimensions. We were interested in each other as people, parents, and artists. I dubbed him my compadre, my co-parent, and friend for life.

We still had a multifaceted bond and a desire for each other to thrive. I never felt I owned Hank; he was a free agent. I think this perception allowed our relationship to continue through all the changes.

In the depositions, Hank, Oz, and I were being portrayed as mainly interested in our sex lives over our children's well-being, which was inaccurate. Our children's welfare was a major consideration in our cohabitation. This way, Hank and I each got to be fully present in their lives, and they got to stay in one home. "How is that not better for them?" we asked ourselves. But apparently parental sexuality and taking good care of children were a complete contradiction. The evaluation seemed to be about discerning whether we were exposing our kids to our deviant sexual lifestyle. But of course, all our sex happened behind locked doors after the children were in bed, just as it would in a healthy, traditional family. The truth is, if Hank and I were truly putting sex ahead of our children's interest, a traditional divorce would have suited us *better*. Then we could each have the kids half the time and wild, kinky orgies when the kids weren't around. But this was not our situation or interest.

That we were the ones being evaluated was mindboggling to me, because in this situation I found the poly mindset brilliant. My kids continued to have parents who loved each other and loved them. And although even people in the poly community might *not* consider what I was doing as poly—because Hank and I were no longer sexual—I did. For me poly was still getting to love Hank and have him close. It wasn't just about a custody arrangement whereby Hank and I lived in a duplex to share the kids. I loved Hank and wanted to maintain our connection. Especially after opening our marriage and dating again, I knew that the love I had with Hank was rare, deep, and inspiring. I still valued it, even though it was a platonic love. That my emotional poly living arrangement caused a huge court battle astonished me.

Oz also had wanted to continue a loving relationship with Susan, although now in the face of the court battle, he was wondering what the basis of their love had been. I became fascinated by how so many people saw divorce—that is, trashing your former spouse—as a "normal" part of a breakup, by how so many people felt that the possibility of transforming the relationship with kindness and grace—still loving each other—was beyond imaginable.

But the court battle did not diminish Oz's wish to keep fighting for a situation that was mainly benefiting me, Hank, and our kids. Oz never asked me to move out with him. He would say, "It just seems preposterous that because you and Hank still like each other we are going to court. The fact that people see that as wrong means that there's something really twisted about our world. You and Hank are doing it in a better way." This sweetness inspired me to dig in all over again and do everything I could to win.

We spent weeks setting up Liam and Amy's rooms in preparation for Edna the Evaluator's tour of the house. We bought Merlin and Liam bunk beds. The week before Edna's scheduled visit Oz took the kids to the zoo, while I spent the entire day cleaning the house and working with a friend putting the finishing touches on the kids' bedrooms. We ironed curtains, bought and assembled furniture. I insisted that we make the rooms perfect.

That evening, Merlin asked to talk to me. He took me into his room with the new bunk beds. Merlin made me lean down so he could whisper in my ear. It was almost as if he was concerned someone would overhear our conversation.

"Mom," Merlin asked, "When will the judge let Liam and Amy sleep over?"

I did my best to explain the situation, that this was a family judge. We hadn't done anything wrong and nobody was going to jail. I could not tell if Merlin was reassured. The whole situation was confusing for him.

Liam never discussed the fact that he couldn't sleep over. At first he was excited about moving in and having sleepovers with Merlin three times a week. But when the court battle started, he stopped talking about it entirely. But that week before Edna's scheduled visit, I was putting dinner on the table, when Liam held up a green cup.

"Gracie, when I move in I want this to be my cup."

I wanted to make sure he felt welcome, so I got my label maker.

"Liam, this is your cup. I'll put your name on it."

Then all the kids insisted that I label their cups, their beds, their bureaus, their doors—it turned into one big label-making party.

The Saturday morning of Edna's visit my hands were shaking as I pulled the pumpkin muffins out of the oven. Oz said he wasn't nervous. But I think he was in his default repress-emotions mode. How could you not be nervous? It was game time and our life hung in the balance!

But when the doorbell rang, I felt an unexpected rush of confidence. Like a prizefighter entering the ring, I opened my front door. My first impression of Edna the Evaluator was that her hair resembled a helmet—a tight bonnet of blond frizz. I was concerned that someone sitting in judgment of our lives had such bad judgment about her hair. But she oozed charm, which both calmed me and made me uneasy. We ate the muffins. I made her an espresso. Edna commented that her coffee was "too hot." So I put a small ice cube in her cup.

We toured my side of the house. Oz had gone to get Liam and Amy, who were required to be there so Edna could watch us interacting. When they returned, Amy crawled into my lap. Liam initiated a spontaneous staring contest with me. Then Amy, Merlin, and Liam ran off playing, while Tallulah stayed close by, observing Edna.

Edna was almost apologetic touring Hank and Valerie's side of the house. I went to bring her up the spiral staircase to their bedroom and she said, "Oh, I don't want to invade your house!"

I said, "Please, invade our house!" and showed her their upstairs bedroom and living room. My thinking was it was intrusive enough to have our home inspected. I wanted her to be thorough so there'd be no excuse to come back again. I hoped her demure attitude was evidence of a forthcoming positive ruling for our team. Edna left after an hour. Then Oz and I had to rush our kids to their respective activities. We talked later by phone and realized we were both completely wiped out. Oz decided to go back to his apartment for an early night with his kids.

I wanted to get a good night's sleep because the next day I was scheduled to meet alone with Edna at her office. But at nine p.m. Oz called me. He could barely talk. When I asked him what was going on he groaned. Apparently, Oz and Susan's nanny had written a character assessment of Oz and submitted it to Edna. Oz considered the nanny somewhat of a friend. But I had never felt good about this woman and had warned Oz about her. Her statements to the court confirmed my suspicions.

Oz read me his copy of the deposition. The nanny described Oz having ropes on his bed. But the only rope Oz had was a thick one under his bed to help his children escape the apartment if there were ever a fire. She mentioned sex toys she found in the closet, along with a poly leaflet. I wondered, again, if it was against the law to experience carnal pleasure? It seemed to be stated as a clear indictment of Oz's character. *He's getting laid! Handcuff him and cart him away!* There were also statements about Oz's apartment being a mess and descriptions of the nanny getting calls from Oz to buy groceries because there was no food in the house. But this was why Oz hired her, to pick up food, laundry detergent, and other household essentials.

But the worst part was a description of Oz dropping his towel and grinning at the nanny. I asked Oz about it because the nanny wasn't his type, as far as I could tell. Oz said he had hired her in the early mornings to help get the kids off to school. The kids were running in and out of his bedroom while he dressed, and the nanny was following them. He'd remembered a moment when his towel briefly slipped, and he had smiled with embarrassment. Nonetheless, the damage was done—the picture painted of Oz was of a filthy, careless, scatter-brained, lecherous creep. Aside from that, he sounded like a great dad.

I tried to rally Oz's spirits but the viciousness of the attack was like a punch in his gut. He was afraid to go to sleep for fear of another nightmare. The past few weeks he'd had a recurring dream of walking down a dark passageway. He would sense a scary presence close by. I decided to help Oz exorcise his demon that night.

"Describe the presence to me."

"It's too amorphous and big to define."

"What is it saying? What does it look like?"

There was a long pause on the other end of the phone. Then Oz groaned.

"What?" I asked.

"It's me. And it's saying: 'You left your family and you deserve to lose your kids.'"

We both went silent.

Then Oz spoke, "Lately I've been afraid that someday I'll regret leaving. What if you and I aren't worth it? What if it costs me my kids?"

Though an unlikely scenario, Edna the Evaluator had the power to recommend Oz get a greatly reduced custody schedule. Also, if the evaluation went badly, Susan could use it in her divorce proceedings to get primary custody or alter visitation to greatly reduce Oz's time with their children. If she got primary custody she could move the children out of state to be closer to her parents, something she'd stated she was interested in doing. All of these scenarios were potential nightmares.

I reassured Oz that this was unlikely. But my words sounded like murmurs in a brash storm. We had to say good night; I needed sleep for the next day. After hanging up, I wandered through the house, drinking chamomile tea and trying to soothe my nerves.

I ran into Hank in the upstairs hall.

"What's up?" he asked. "You look awful."

"Thanks!" I replied, then told Hank what the nanny had written. "Now Oz is worried our relationship won't be worth it. I hate this evaluation."

"He's grieving what his marriage could have been, not what it actually was," Hank said. "Your boy is hurting. I've seen him staring off into space, and I know he's worrying about losing his kids."

"I know, I know."

We were in what used to be our bedroom. Hank was sitting on the stool in front of my vanity; I was on the California king bed that felt like my life raft. I sipped my tea.

I said, "Do you remember when we visited my dad? Remember when Angela told us about my dad's depression after he and my mom divorced?"

When I was twenty-six, Hank encouraged me to reunite with my dad when he discovered how much I was struggling with my daddy issues. My stepmother cried when she described my parent's divorce, imploring me not to keep asking my father about why I never saw him as a child.

"I hated that my dad never fought for me," I admitted. "But watching what Oz is going through makes me think of my dad in a different light. I don't think he had the resources financially or emotionally for this kind of a battle."

Hank's eyes were moist. "Maybe that's why your father wouldn't do therapy with you when you asked him. Maybe he couldn't open up that dark place where he knew he didn't have the strength to fight for you."

We were both crying. I started making involuntary snorting noises, and spontaneously we started laughing. I shook my head.

"I can't believe I actually feel compassion for my dad. I guess I should be grateful for this lovely gift."

"Like a flower blossoming in a cesspool," Hank said, and we giggled. "Is everything okay with you and Oz?"

"Yes, I think we make a good…" I couldn't think of the word to use in front of my husband; there was one on the tip of my tongue but I didn't want to go there.

"Couple?" Hank offered, raising an eyebrow.

"Yes! That was the word I was searching for."

It felt a bit odd telling my husband that Oz and I worked as a couple. We bid each other good night.

The next morning, although tired, I entered my appointment with confidence. I still felt that once I talked with Edna directly she'd understand what we were doing. I sat down on a thin couch.

Edna started asking a series of questions that made me wonder if she thought poly was an irresponsible, selfish lifestyle. I was a bit stunned by the candid bigotry. I explained that people who did poly well had really happy partners and an ability to tune in to their mates, listen, and respond. She asked about Valerie, who had been at a dance class when she visited our home. Edna assumed Valerie was in her twenties—Valerie was forty. *Where did she get that?* I wondered.

She asked about how I met Oz, and I explained the three-year odyssey, culminating with me opening my marriage. Then her cell phone rang, and she answered it. There was a brief discussion with someone. Edna hung up and announced the session was over. She had to lend her daughter her car. I was somewhat shocked by the unprofessionalism. I had wanted to talk further, even ask some questions of my own.

But walking to my car, it hit me. This was the perfect job for a mediocre therapist. There was a hefty fee upfront, and you could procrastinate and overbook clients. Most important, the people who paid you could not voice any complaints about you, for fear of getting a bad evaluation.

I drove home slowly contemplating what to say to Oz. I had a sick feeling in my gut. When I got home Oz was waiting. I wanted to be a source of optimism, but I had to share my fears. Until now I had banked on Edna the Evaluator being a reasonable, unbigoted person who had intelligence and an open mind. Now I could see that was a hope we could not depend on. We discussed quietly what we would do if we could never live together full-time.

"My home is here with you," Oz said. "If I am forced to live in two places it will be like not having a home. If I lose that opportunity I'll never be whole again."

Oz started to cry. I watched him. I felt like John Wayne, watching his costar weep while I scratched around for solutions. I bit my lip so hard it hurt. I got Oz into this. I had to get us through it. One thing was for sure—we could not depend on the court system to be fair. We had to find a way to take our power back.

Chapter 19

After my meeting with Edna the Evaluator, we contacted Oz's lawyer and voiced our concerns. She reassured us that we were overreacting and that most people felt "picked on" during an evaluation. Over the next few weeks the evaluation seemed to be stalled to almost a complete halt. Finally, we demanded that our lawyer do something. She called and e-mailed Edna several times but got no response.

Finally our lawyer got Edna on the phone while she was driving. She probably answered by mistake. Edna said she would be done with the evaluation the first week of October; it was now June!

Our lawyer called us later and said, "The evaluator has all the power here and we don't want to offend her. Let's just wait till October."

The next day Oz came to my house with a grievance. He said that the day before Amy had had a fever. Because he didn't want to take her out of his apartment, he and Liam had been trapped inside while Amy slept. Oz felt complete frustration. He reasoned that if we lived together, he could have taken Merlin and Liam on an adventure while I took care of Amy and hung out with Tallulah—a simple division of labor that would've pleased everyone.

"I want to give up my apartment. It has come to represent everything I hate about my life."

"Can you do that?"

"I don't care. I am sick of waiting for this evaluation to be done."

"Where would you sleep on the nights you have your kids?"

"What if I found an inexpensive studio apartment—just a bedroom for me, Amy, and Liam? We could spend every waking hour here, then sleep at the apartment."

"But how will this affect the evaluation?"

Oz shook his head, "I don't know."

We pulled out a yellow legal pad and listed all the pros and cons. The pro to keeping the apartment was that it was a stable situation until the evaluation was over. The con was that it was an expensive burden that isolated Oz, making it harder to coparent together. We called Oz's lawyer, who cautioned Oz not to do it. Oz hung up.

"What does it matter, the pros and cons? I just can't do it anymore."

I could have continued to counsel Oz to remain stable, as our lawyer warned, but there was a way that this new move was appealing. The point of the court hearings were to attempt to prevent us from becoming a family—which was already happening. We had been playing to the courts, to the judge, to the evaluator—*what if we did something proactive?* It felt right.

That week we toured a few small apartments—nothing was quite right. I asked all my friends if they knew of any studios for lease, when Freya suggested her flat. She had a separate section that wasn't being used. Oz toured her apartment and gave her a check on the spot. At the end of the month we moved everything into my house except the bare minimum for Freya's apartment, which became like a small locker in which you kept your towels at the beach. Both lawyers were not happy with the situation. But Oz told his lawyer, "I heard your advice and I don't agree with it." We were sick of lawyers, sick of the evaluation.

After the switch, our lives improved. We made dinners together. Even though the kids could not sleep over, they moved all their toys and clothes into their new rooms. We were starting to think outside the lines in terms of our little tribe. We were in a determined cycle of taking back our power. If the courts ruled against us and the kids could never sleep over, we'd come up with some new creative solution—they could not prevent us from becoming a family.

I felt both zealous and overwhelmed by the blending of all our personalities. The younger three children loved to play together, so on Saturdays Oz frequently took them to the park, the zoo, or the jumpy house emporium. Merlin loved Oz's massive playful energy.

But around this time, Merlin began having small tantrums. Whenever Oz was in the mix, Merlin behaved like a displaced ape in the land of the big-boy apes. Both Merlin and Oz were alpha males. They had fun together but also competed. When Merlin's behavior was baffling me, Oz turned out to be a surprising resource. One night I tried to get Merlin to brush his teeth—thoroughly, in a way that would not entail more money to the dentist. I stood overseeing operations. Merlin was getting angrier by the minute.

Finally Oz pulled me aside.

"Merlin feels insulted."

"What?" Could motherhood get any more confusing?

"It would be better if you said, 'Merlin, show me how fantastic you are at brushing your teeth.' Merlin feels like you are telling him he doesn't know how to brush his teeth."

I followed Oz's directions, practically speaking in a Scarlett O'Hara drawl—and it worked. Merlin almost flexed his little biceps as he brushed under my adoring gaze.

But a few weeks later we had another meltdown. After dinner, Tallulah, Oz, Merlin, and I were playing cards. When Merlin lost to Oz, he cried, "Oz cheated!" This was his frequent lament when he lost to Oz, who refused to run slower or feign weakness so Merlin could win. Oz felt "fake losing" would be a worse insult to Merlin. The situation was exhausting. After some gladiator battle—racing to the car or shooting hoops—Merlin would collapse into a ball of tears. Then Merlin and Oz would lock horns like two moose in the forest, both stubborn, both annoying.

Merlin starting sobbing, "Oz always wins. It isn't fair!" This wrenched my heart. Oz and I spent many nights discussing the situation late at night behind closed doors. I asked him how he handled competing with Liam. But Liam had no interest in sports or competition, so this was new territory for Oz. I asked Oz how this was handled in his family of origin. He described a bunch of cutthroat big brains vying to win. My heart sank.

Then one night, Oz and Merlin were arm wrestling at the dining room table. I challenged Tallulah, while Merlin took Oz on. Merlin managed to hold on for few moments; then Oz pinned his hand down and Merlin sat crying. I was exhausted at the thought of another go-round. Tallulah and I told Merlin that Oz was more than one hundred pounds heavier. *How could Merlin possibly win?*

Our logic further angered Merlin, who ranted, "Oz cheated!"

I wondered, *What did he really feel Oz had cheated him out of?*

Oz sat quietly. Tallulah and I fell into a perplexed silence. The only sound in the room was Merlin's choked sobs. I was contemplating what to do next when Oz leaned into Merlin.

"It's okay, Merlin," Oz said. "In about twelve years you'll kick my ass at arm wrestling."

Merlin's tears stopped, and he looked up at Oz.

In his raspy little voice he repeated, "In twelve years I am going to kick your ass?"

We all laughed at the sudden change in Merlin's demeanor.

Oz continued, "Oh, yes. I'll be fifty, you'll be eighteen—you'll kick my ass. You'll be stronger than me."

Merlin slowly grinned. He saw the dawn of a new age—an age in which he'd be the dominant male. Amazingly, from this point on, Merlin's relationship with Oz shifted. They relaxed with each other. I put a basketball hoop in the side yard. After dinner, Oz and Merlin would go outside and play basketball. As I sipped my wine, I'd hear Oz yell, "I am going to win, Little Man!" Merlin would erupt with laughter, then get a basket. Oz would yell, "You are going down, Little Man! You are going down." But it was all okay, now that Merlin understood who was really going down.

I felt triumphant when things fell into place. But the nights Oz spent away with his kids, I would often wake up in the darkest hours, my heart beating anxiously over the possibility that we might never be allowed to all live under one roof as a family.

One evening after dropping off Liam and Amy, Oz sat down at our counter.

"I am going to call Susan and see if we can't work something out," he said.

"What?"

I was making Oz's new favorite drink. I loathed the omen-like quality of Oz's usual drink, the Dark and Stormy. At one of our favorite restaurants we both tasted a citrusy cocktail that with each sip imbued a person with a feeling of sun and smooth sailing. It contained rye, bitters, a fresh orange, and Amaro. Because I couldn't think of an easy solution to our troubles, I had resorted to encouraging Oz to drink more.

As I poured the elixir from the shaker of crushed ice, I asked, "So, you're just going to call her?"

"This evaluation is taking far too long. Perhaps there's a way to both get what we want."

I nodded, but internally I had serious doubts. It just seemed ludicrous to call Susan after months of court drama. I voiced my trepidation. But Oz carried his drink outside. He reclined on our bamboo lounge chair, took a sip from his martini glass, and pulled out his cell. I watched him from the kitchen as I sliced vegetables. Forty-five minutes later Oz came back in. He set down his glass.

"She's open to talking."

I refilled his glass. I didn't think it was going to work. But besides drinking, I didn't have a better solution, so I remained silent. For the next several days I would gaze out of my picture window to the side yard where Oz was quietly talking on his cell phone. The conversations went on for hours. Sometimes I would step outside and hear Oz saying things like, "I can't agree to that, but let's figure out another scenario that will work for both of us." I was impressed that he wasn't screaming at her after everything that had been said about him in the depositions.

Five days later I was shaving my legs in the bathtub when Oz walked in.

"Susan has agreed to let the kids move in if I give up Monday nights."

"What?" I nearly sliced my ankle with my razor. "How did you do that?"

"I think she wants control back over her life as much as we do. Also, her lawyers might be telling her that she's going to lose," Oz shrugged. "I didn't tell her my lawyers were warning me that I might lose."

I obsessively interrogated Oz for the next thirty minutes and the next several days. What changed? What made her agree to this when she was so opposed to the kids living in my home?

The whole situation was so painful for him that our discussions frequently ended with Oz saying, "Let's just move on."

Move on we did. Oz's chagrined lawyers (who ultimately had contributed very little to resolving the dispute and helping us win our case) e-mailed custody documents for Oz and Susan to sign. We had asked them to hurry, lest Susan change her mind. The lawyers hammered out a set of legal agreements that basically amounted to allowing the kids to live with us until the final ruling in October. When they arrived via e-mail, Oz immediately signed and sent them to Susan for her signature.

We were ecstatic. We took the rest of the day off. I put on a crimson minidress with leopard high heels and Oz and I set out for University Avenue to celebrate. We got wine, a beet salad, and polenta. Then we picked up the kids from school and brought them to our favorite Italian restaurant. Oz choked up when we told them they could sleep over this weekend.

After we got the okay to move the kids in, we hired a child psychologist to tour our home and give us pointers. Criticized repeatedly, we were scared that we might have missed something crucial, so we thought this was a good idea. The psychologist arrived at the appointed hour and immediately toured our side of the house. We explained the living arrangement: the kids are free to go to either side of the duplex at any time, and adults respect good boundaries by knocking or calling. Then I showed her Hank and Valerie's side.

At the end of the tour, she asked us if we'd heard about "nesting." I had not heard of the term, and neither had Oz. Apparently, nesting was a situation whereby a divorced couple took turns being in the family home, where the kids lived permanently, so that the children never had to switch houses.

"I've never seen anyone do this," she said quietly. "This is better than nesting. Your children have access to both you and their father twenty-four hours a day, seven days a week. Fantastic job." Then I walked her out and shut the door. Oz and I stood like statues for a second.

Then I whispered, "Did you hear what she said...*fantastic job...?*"

We clasped hands, giggling.

"Baby!" I said. "Somebody just told us we're doing it right!"

After months of being examined with suspicion, a certified "child expert" had affirmed what we believed—that we were moving through a huge life change gracefully and with our children's well-being foremost in our minds. We were pioneers.

In October, we got Edna the Evaluator's report. Our lawyer called Oz to deliver the news—Edna had allowed the kids to permanently live in our house—we had won! Our lawyer told us she'd only read the conclusion—which contained Edna's recommendation to the judge.

"Congratulations, sounds like Edna really liked you."

She e-mailed over the evaluation saying she'd call back after reading it. We began scrutinizing the report. After a few pages I got a queasy feeling in my gut—reading the report felt like getting a severe spanking from the status quo. Oz's lawyer called back ten minutes later.

"Guess I spoke a little too quickly about Edna liking you."

"Do her statements have any weight beyond the conclusion?" Oz asked.

Our lawyer reassured us that it didn't matter if the evaluator disapproved of our alternative lifestyle, as long as the final conclusion said the kids could live with us.

After reading the report for an hour it felt to me like really bad reality TV with obvious clichés. If producers ever got hold of our story, I'd surely be edited to look like that predictably bitchy diva reigning with supreme power over her men and the household. This was exactly the stereotype I had originally feared people would make about me when we embarked upon our alternative lifestyle. In my opinion, this was the level of sophistication in the report.

I took a deep breath and forced myself to step away from Oz's computer. Oz slumped in his chair, drained. When I took a moment to scan my body, I realized I was shaking. But instead of stilling myself, I felt an overwhelming need to move. I got up to see if any of the kids wanted to go on a walk to get ice cream. *Let's overeat!* Liam, Amy, and Merlin were building a fort, but Tallulah was up for a walk.

We stepped onto the sidewalk and headed down the street. Oz texted me—still shaken by the idea that the courts had so much power over our lives. I texted him back and then put my phone away. Down on the avenue pedestrians bustled by us; I could feel a knot in my shoulders undoing itself. But even though we'd won, I still felt shell shocked. It didn't feel like justice had been served; rather, it felt like we had barely squeaked by, and mainly due to Oz's negotiating ingenuity and money. I couldn't help but wonder about other, more vulnerable families.

Tallulah and I kept walking toward the ice cream shop; I was thankful it was a long hike. With each step I felt more solid. The moon was huge—a golden harvest moon. At the beginning of our walk I could barely see it between the trees, but as we got closer to downtown it seemed to have elevated itself above all else—giving the night an otherworldly splendor. It gazed back at me, like an old friend watching me through all my travails, a steady presence that soothed me. We sat down on a bench with our ice cream cones. I put my hand over my heart, my own touch calming me. *We did it, and we won,* I said quietly to myself like a mantra. The realization swept over me, and I suddenly felt like I was holding a silver ray of moonlight in my pocket.

But there were a new set of challenges. Was it just me or had the volume exponentially increased? Oz's kids were *loud.* It wasn't just shouting and playing; it was video games with constant explosions and the TV with the volume turned up. I cooked dinner in what sounded like a napalmed stretch of war zone. I talked to Hank about it one afternoon. Our kids just seemed genetically quieter. But Hank reminded me of a piece of real estate we'd bought near a highway. After escrow closed we stood in the backyard, where I noticed the harsh traffic noise for the first time.

"I didn't notice how loud the traffic was before."

"We didn't own it before."

Now I owned the whole package: Oz and kids in tow. Luckily, Oz was a wizard at solving practical problems. The next day he came home with laptops for Tallulah and Liam and two smaller devices for Merlin and Amy—and four sets of earphones. The kids plugged in and Oz took down our huge flat-screen TV. That night I cooked dinner soothed by the sweet sound of quiet.

But there was also the massive uptick in clutter. Had Oz gotten messier right after the evaluation? Like a giant belch of relief his clothes were strewn all over our bedroom. And he hadn't been picking up after his kids. I reassured myself that this was a temporary glitch.

Having routines helped order the chaos. My favorite was meeting up with Oz in our room after we'd put our kids to bed at nine p.m. One Friday night, two months after the court ruling, I was waiting in my pink negligee with a freshly (that very afternoon!) waxed pussy. Things ran late with Oz's kids and I fell asleep. Early the next morning behind locked bedroom doors, I dangled the freshly waxed pussy over Oz's mouth—just as we heard Amy coming down the stairs.

Feeling defeated but determined to be a good sport, I got up and started baking Saturday-morning muffins, another routine. It was there, in the kitchen—while mixing the batter to the soundtrack of blasting cartoons, and while the promise of a new round of dirty dishes and messy living room mocked my vision of a kick-back weekend—that the exuberance over the court "win" was deflated like a sad balloon after the birthday party. Had I created a situation in which I'd be engulfed by more domestic duties and less passion? After the muffins came out of the oven, I called a friend practically panting with anxiety.

"For over a year I've been fighting for more children to move in. Why didn't you pimp-slap some sense into me?" I told my friend. "Have I just replicated my marriage problems all over again?"

But at our VHOG that week we discussed the kids' adjustment issues at length, then aligned calendars for our romantic weekends away. It was very clear we had a unified vision: we wanted the kids to thrive and we wanted time for ourselves. My nerves were soothed on that front.

But housework and parenting styles proved to be two areas where we had to repeatedly hammer out agreements. The dishwasher, as magnificent as it was, could not load itself. Oz, with his engineering mind, was remarkably good at creating "cleaning systems." Over time we trained our children to help with chores. I began to understand how large families with eight or nine kids could function without total mayhem.

Life started to normalize, and I felt good again about what we had created. In that first year we worked on dynamics of our new family and co-parenting. Congruently, Oz and I were adjusting to being full-time partners. I was apprehensive that in our domesticity we'd become nonsexual. Especially when even a freshly waxed pussy couldn't override our exhaustion or the kids' needs. It did help that Oz was crazy horny. He was up for a quickie midday, then another serving at night. The first several months I never turned down an opportunity to get me some. After a year of living together, I was afforded the luxury of occasionally playing hard to get. A few times when I had six a.m. clients and Oz started rubbing on me at midnight, I had to inform him "the kitchen is closed." But Oz was an ardent pursuer who would do almost anything to wake up my libido, and he usually succeeded in getting a late-night snack.

I loved the vast playground we'd created erotically: shadow sex, playful sex, competitive sex. We were doing so many things in bed that I'd once considered as a feminist to be taboo. But I was still stymied with the ass project. One night I decided to let go of my vigilant internal feminist and follow what really turned me on—in hopes I'd bypass my tight ass. I told Oz my masturbation fantasy—the king and the village girl—embarrassingly cliché yet so hot. Oz (as the king) would select me out of all the other succulent village girls. It was a Harlequin romance on steroids—so far off the feminist grid it made me cringe. Oz loved it; after all the village girl was willing to do *anything* to please and satisfy her king.

With my ass in the air, Oz caressed my rosebud. Oz told me he wanted to put his cock up my ass and that this would distinguish me from all the other village girls. He started to finger me. I let myself be opened, but when he edged his cock in *I just could not do it.* The angle felt dangerously vulnerable.

We decided to try missionary. Something about the eye contact made me feel more in control. I placed Oz at my anus and he started to edge in. We got to the impasse—my sphincter tightened against the intrusion. I was crushed that it wasn't going to work yet again. But Oz stepped into the role of the omnipotent yet benevolent King.

He whispered, "Let me just stay here." He had only penetrated me about an inch.

We looked into each other's eyes, and it was both the most intimate moment and the kinkiest moment I'd ever experienced. We gazed at each other. Oz would not back down.

"Let me in," he commanded, spoken in the sweetest, ever-loving, ever-strong tone. I took a deep breath and felt myself open another centimeter.

Oz moved deeper inside me. "Give yourself to me."

I opened a bit more.

"I love you so much, Gracie."

We were breathing in unison. It was unbearably sexy to feel so owned and possessed. Then I asked that he pull out just a tad. He did, and somehow his retreat made it possible for me to open more. He plunged forward, now almost completely inside me.

"It's just a little more," he whispered, "give it to me, give me your ass."

The final thrust was surprisingly the easiest. He was suddenly fully inside me. It was both a shock and the sweetest moment of pleasure. He moved within me carefully; I could not handle any deep pounding. His satisfied surprise to have fully possessed me made him moan with pleasure. I moaned too; having Oz in my ass was so different than having him inside my pussy. My pussy was a friendly, easy, plush ride. But my ass was like a tightrope, a triumph to control and not plunge to your death. I felt fragile; one wrong pounding of Oz's deep, muscular thighs and I'd tear.

There were so many more nerve endings, thousands of them bundled together ready to burst with each thrust; there was fear and pleasure at the same time. Within moments I came so forcefully and so quickly that I had to push Oz out of me. He rolled over on the bed and collapsed. We lay next to each other moaning again and again. I was stunned that ecstasy had entered my mundane life through the backdoor.

For so many years I had been riding on a vague sense that sex, joy, and pleasure could be healing. A trite New Age book I'd once read implored to "learn through joy." The idea appealed to me, but I had to admit some of my greatest teachers had been the pain in my root chakra, pain from loss, pain from life—generalized, ongoing angst that became my engine of change as it sought its natural counterpart, joy. I realized that this was what happened in my lovemaking with Oz—my pain was literally flipped on its ass. Pain is the shadow of pleasure, and if you have the courage to feel both, ecstasy awaits you. With the healing presence of love, there is no place in our hearts or minds—or asses—that is untouchable.

I usually approached Christmas like a beggar. Every year it was a crisis. The holidays were a reminder of my lack of an extended family. I would practically put a gun to my brother's head, demanding his presence on Christmas morning. I wore out therapists on the subject. Around November, Judy would get a look of dread in her eyes.

Finally Reenie advised me, "Just think of it as a quiet day with your family."

And that helped immensely. I forced myself to lower my expectations.

That year, with Oz, Valerie, Liam, and Amy, we numbered eight—then nine when my brother showed up, and twelve when Merlin's pal Phoenix arrived in the late afternoon with his dad and stepmom for martinis and Monopoly. I was ecstatic, making lasagna and white clam sauce linguini. The kids opened their presents and played in their pajamas for the entire morning—it was bustling.

There was a moment in this new-fangled Norman Rockwell Christmas that will forever be emblazoned in my mind. Merlin and Phoenix were taking turns swinging on the climbing rope we'd attached to the twenty-foot ceilings in the middle of our living room. Merlin gave the rope to Phoenix and ran upstairs to get gloves. While I went into the room to try to salvage my couch pillows that Amy, Merlin, and Phoenix had built into a fort, Phoenix swung by me. I liked this kid and took an instant liking to his parents, who were both sculptors. They had separated when Phoenix was a baby but were still good friends and had lofts a good thirty minutes from each other.

"You have the coolest house!" Phoenix said. The kid was an electric jolt of energy.

"Thanks," I replied as I assembled my pillows back on the couch.

Phoenix leaped off the swing and landed next to me. "You know why?"

"Why?"

"It has gigantic windows, and you have a rope swing in the middle of your living room. But the best thing of all is that Merlin gets to have both his mom and his dad whenever he wants them!"

I almost started crying. My kids hadn't mentioned our arrangement in months—it was now so commonplace to them. Judy reassured me that this was a good thing. They had acclimated. I went off to get a tissue at my desk and absentmindedly started shuffling through some photos I'd taken two years ago when we started this whole crazy ride.

There was a picture I took of Oz and Hank looking up at me from the roadster Oz brought home from work that weekend. Hank squinted into the sun with a seasoned, wise expression; Oz was smiling, both jaunty and unbearably handsome. But what moved me so was that both of them were gazing at me with such love.

I remember visiting Hoover Dam one summer with Hank. I was struck by the massive achievement of 6.6 million tons of concrete. I could imagine what the engineers and workers went through planning and then executing the construction: it would be a monstrously difficult achievement, but by gum, where there's a will, there's a way.

If someone had told me five years ago, "You are going to have Oz and still keep everything you love, Hank, and the happy family you've created," I would have thought she was nuts. I could see how this transformation could become like Hoover Dam, cars passing it every day, a commonplace landmark but still an outlandishly spectacular accomplishment. I had achieved my dream, my version of poly, my unique family.

I felt infinitely blessed.

Epilogue

When I look back at the time period in which *Wide Open* took place, I am filled with gratitude that Valerie, Oz, Hank, and I were willing and able to be relationship innovators and do something different. Hank and Valerie lived in the duplex for about four years, and then they decided to move to have their own place a few miles away. I still love Hank immensely and consider him family.

There is an evolution happening in marriage and long-term relationships whereby people are creating unique agreements with their partners. There is no correct way to do it; in fact, I believe we are all on a spectrum, and make many nuanced choices that span from monogamy to polyamory. No one size fits all, and each of us has our own unique relationship ideology. To me, the ultimate outcome I desire in this current evolution is having relationships that can contain more of who we are, build more trust and passion, and allow for fluidity and change so that we may grow together versus apart. To that end, I am eternally grateful for my relationship odyssey that took place over these past years.

Namaste,

Gracie X

Acknowledgments

This book started off as a casual journal, first as aversion therapy to overcome my love for Oz and then as my own fascinated notes when I leaped off a cliff and opened my marriage. It swelled up to more than four hundred pages, which I was wading through when the Goddess of Destiny sent to my Pilates gym the earthbound publishing Goddess Catharine Sutker Meyers. After six months of roll-ups and pelvic-floor strengthening, I began regaling her with stories about polyamory and dating while married. I told her I was writing a book on the subject, and she asked to see a few pages. Her wisdom and vision, continually steering me to the deeper themes of the material, have been invaluable. Catharine, I thank you many times over—you truly championed this book.

I extend a huge thank-you to my New Harbinger editors: Jess Beebe, Melissa Valentine, and Nicola Skidmore. Your intelligence, searing observations, and almost eerie ability to ferret out revisionist passages have vastly improved my book. Marisa Solís, your final edits took the book to a whole new level; my gratitude for your "Marisa magic" is immense.

Great thanks to the New Harbinger dream team that rallied around my book in the final hours. Matt McKay, Catharine Sutker Meyers (yet again), Jonathan Kirsch, Troy DuFrene, and Heather Garnos. And to Andy P. for her support in all ways to get my book through its final passage.

I thank Dave Eaton for his skillful promotions; my brother, David, and sister, Tina, for the inspiration to be stronger and not just survive but thrive; and my coven sisters, the Mavens, who always give me courage to dream big and work magically with any obstacles, and who are all warriors in the service of love.

Great thanks goes to my many invaluable friends: Maureen Claussen, for her emotional intelligence and willingness to laugh hard; Kaila Flexor, for her wry humor and wisdom; Kate Shaheed, for long talks on the nature of loving and alternative relationship structures; Kelly Manashil, for her humor and quick understanding of what I was trying to achieve; and Liyana Silver, for her brilliance and forward thinking. Endless thanks to Lydia Adkins and Meagan Radowski, for being warriors and seekers who helped me explore the vast possibilities and openings to more love; Judy Jones, for significant turning-point breakthroughs in how to structure relationship and family; Johanna Self, for wise council on child development and blended family; and Sarah Corr, for reading and copyediting the book many times over, and for her shrewd advice on the book and in all areas of my life.

Finally, always great thanks to Hank, for his dedication to love, art, family, progressive thinking, and living creatively. Also to Valerie, for being willing to do something different and for the hours of processing and the deep love shared with my kids.

Oddly, I am inspired to acknowledge my mother, now long dead. But somehow as I write these acknowledgments at three a.m. in the witching hour and darkness of the night, I can hear her strong voice urging me on. If nothing else, you blessed me with buckets of gumption.

To my children, who inspire me every day to be a stronger, better person, and to Oz, who read, edited, engineered, continually shored me up as I wrote, and repeatedly resolved all technical and life problems through graphs, logic, passion, and much intelligence. Oz, you inspired this book a thousand times over. I thank you.

WIDE OPEN

DISCUSSION GUIDE

1. Discuss how Gracie's feelings about her marriage and sex life made her feel (before she opened her marriage). Have you ever met a person like Gracie who talks openly about her need for sex? Does talking about this make you feel uncomfortable, or do you enjoy talking openly about sex?

2. Does Gracie—in her forties when the events of the book take place, and in her fifties now—seem like a typical middle-aged woman to you? Do you relate to her anxieties? Do you relate to her confidence and boldness?

3. Do you think Gracie would have asked for an open marriage if she had never met Oz?

4. Would it offend, hurt, or excite you if your partner asked if you would be game to have an open relationship? Do you know anyone in an open marriage? What are your thoughts about those who live polyamorously?

5. When Tallulah, Gracie's daughter, finds out about the relationship between Gracie and her "special friend" Oz, she is shaken. How do you think the relationships between Gracie, Oz, Hank, and Valerie affect their children? How do you think it would affect your children?

6. What do you think Gracie saw in Oz that made her want him sexually? Lust, love, or a way out of an unhappy marriage?

7. Do you believe that Gracie caused the end of Oz's marriage to Susan, or do you believe it was inevitable?

8. Do you think you have a more positive view of poly relationships after reading this book, or are you more distrustful of them?

9. Do you believe that lust and love are separate drives? Or do you need both for a happy marriage?

10. Are the anal sex scenes between Oz and Gracie motivated more by lust, love, or a combination of both?

11. When Aurora, Gracie's poly counselor, tells Gracie and Hank that they aren't poly, Gracie wonders if she's just traded one set of rules for another. Describe the implicit and explicit rules you have in your relationship. If you could change one of those rules, which would it be?

12. What is strikingly out of the norm in Oz and Hank's relationship, and in Valerie and Gracie's?

13. Toward the end of the book, Gracie says she is living a different kind of Norman Rockwell painting and loving it. Do you think Gracie and Hank would ever have been able to achieve this happiness on their own? If you were to open your own relationship, do you think it would survive? What might jeopardize it (jealousy, trust issues)?

14. If you could ask Gracie a question personally, what would it be? Same goes for Hank, Oz, and their children.

The *Wide Open* Discussion Guide is also available for free download at https://www.newharbinger.com/openguide

Gracie X is a writer, actress, and director. She lives in Northern California. Find out more about Gracie at http://GracieX.com, and connect with her online:

Facebook: https://www.facebook.com/GracieXauthor

Twitter: https://twitter.com/GracieXauthor

YouTube: https://www.youtube.com/channel/ UCrpUKF87ojhzmV4uVNNyGAA

Foreword writer **Carol Queen, PhD**, cofounded the Center for Sex and Culture in San Francisco with her partner, Robert Morgan Lawrence. Queen is also staff sexologist at Good Vibrations, and author of *Real Live Nude Girl: Chronicles of Sex-Positive Culture*.